Sudoku Puzzles

In sudoku, each row, column and box (spaces of 3 x 3) needs to be filled out with the numbers 1-9, without repeating any within the row, column or box.

The catch is that you can only use each number once – no number can be repeated in a row, column, or box.

Puzzle #1

HARD

		8				7	9	
			7		5			
			4	3		2		
7			6	1			2	
4		1			7	9		
8	2							
9		5	1				7	
					4	5		

Puzzle #2
HARD

5			8		7			
		9		4		5	2	
								7
9							5	
		8						6
	1		2	3			8	
			1					
8		2			6			
	3	1				4		

Puzzle #3

HARD

					2			6
7	8		4					
			3			2	5	
			1	9		5		2
1	6	8						
	2							7
5				4			9	
8	7							
								1

Puzzle #4

HARD

				9				2
4				9				5
		3	7				1	
6	2		3				8	
					5	9		
						1		
	5		2	4	8			
8				6				9
		1				7		

Puzzle #5

HARD

	9			3				
			7		5		2	9
2					6	5	1	7
7					1	8		
	6						3	5
	8							
3		5			7			8
	2		4					6
4								

Puzzle #6

HARD

			6	7				5
9						8		
	1							3
	5	6		8		7		1
			2					6
	8		5	2		3		
		7						
	2		1		3		9	

Puzzle #7

HARD

			2			6	3	
	7						9	
				1	7			
		8						
6		3			8	7		
7				4		1	6	
			3		9			
	3			2				
			8	6				4

Puzzle #8

HARD

				3		4	2	
	1					8	7	
	8			2	1			6
	5			6		9		
6			4	1				
3			5					
8			6		1			
	9			2			6	7

Puzzle #9

HARD

3	6							8
		9			4			
		8				2		5
					1	5	2	4
7		4		6				
				9			3	7
6	4		3	7				
8			9					
2					6			

Puzzle #10

HARD

1	6				3			
			4		6			
	7	4						
	2						7	
5					1		2	
				5				6
8		5		4		1		
7				1	8	6		4
					2			9

Puzzle #11

HARD

		6					9		
1	3				6	4		
		9			3			
6								1
7			5		2		6	
5	4		3					
							8	
			7	8		1		2
			2				5	7

Puzzle #12

HARD

	6							
	8		1					6
3						4		
		2		6		5		
	5		2	9				
				4			7	
4	3							9
								3
	2		7		8			1

Puzzle #13

HARD

5	2				4			
				6				
7						8	2	1
1			3				8	
3	4		6			9		
	8			2	9	7		
9						6	3	
		1					5	
								8

Puzzle #12

HARD

	6							
	8		1					6
3						4		
		2		6		5		
		5	2	9				
				4			7	
4	3							9
								3
	2		7		8			1

Puzzle #13

HARD

5	2				4			
				6				
7						8	2	1
1			3				8	
3	4		6			9		
	8			2	9	7		
9						6	3	
		1					5	
								8

Puzzle #14

HARD

	9				5	6		2
		4					7	3
3			1	7				
		8			1			
5			8					
			4				5	
	6				4			
2			9				1	
1				6			9	5

Puzzle #15

HARD

		6		3	2			1
						9		
	7		8					
4			5	6				
2							9	
				9	8			
3							2	6
7			9				1	
		8	1	5				

Puzzle #16

HARD

			1			6		
		6						
	8	5			3		7	
9	7						4	
				2			6	
		3	8					
		7		6	9	1	3	
	9			1				4
	4		2					

Puzzle #17

HARD

							4	
			2			7		1
		3	4		5	9		2
1			3					
5				6	9	2		
2		9					8	
			1					3
			7	8				

Puzzle #18

HARD

1		7				5		
5			8					
	3	4			7		8	
			2			1	9	
8			4					6
				6				5
				3	9		2	
	4		5			6		1

Puzzle #19

HARD

		4	9					
9					3		7	
	5							8
4							2	7
2				1				
1				5			4	
			4	7		6		
3		9	8					
	6					8		

Puzzle #20

HARD

			7					2
	4	6				1	7	
			5			9		
7	6			4				
9		8						
			1	5	6			
	1					4		
	2				3			
			8				5	1

Puzzle #21

HARD

	4		6				8	1
				8			5	
3		1			9			
							7	
2			9	3				
	5							4
		6	1				4	
	7	4						6
				5			1	

Puzzle #22

HARD

		2					8	
			4				7	3
		9				5		6
				1				8
			6		8	9	4	
3								
8				5		3		
7	5			6				
	6		7		1			

Puzzle #23

HARD

	7			5			9	
		3			6		7	5
		9		1		2		
7		1			8	6		
							3	
8				6	3	4		2
2				3				
			1	4				8

Puzzle #24

HARD

			8					
	4						2	
7	8				6			
				6		8		
	5		2			3		
3				5				1
8	6		4					
			9					
4	5	7	3				6	2

Puzzle #25

HARD

			8		6	9		
		1	3					4
7				4			2	3
	3							8
9						7		
	6		4					2
3					7			5
			2	1	9	8		

Puzzle #26

HARD

			6			8		
7				5				4
	9	6		7				3
					2			7
				4				5
1			7					
	5							
	2		8			1	4	
	3						9	

Puzzle #27

HARD

7			4					
	6	2	8				3	
1		5	2	3			4	
3			1	7	8	4		
				5			7	
	8							6
	4							
			7		1		2	9

Puzzle #28

HARD

		8						
	5							9
	9			6	4			
1					8	2		7
9							1	
		3			2			6
	7		3	1		5	2	
				5			4	
						9		1

Puzzle #29

HARD

				1				
5	6	8		2			1	
	9	1		5		6		2
				3			7	
	8				1			
		9	8			4		
		5			6			
						3	9	5
	1				4		2	

Puzzle #30

HARD

9				3			8	
	8	5					2	
6			7	2		1		
			4			5		
	4			6				
1		8	2				6	
							4	
					1			3
		2		9	6			

Puzzle #31

HARD

4					9	8		7
			6				1	
5								4
	7			1				
	6		7				4	
8		3		2				5
	3			6				
						4		2
			8		5	9		

Puzzle #32

HARD

		3		9				
		5		3	7		1	
					2		4	
		1		5		6		4
	6		1	8		5		
3		7						8
9					5			
7							2	
				1		7		

Puzzle #33

HARD

9			1	2				
			5		9	8		
1			6			4		
	5	1			6	7		9
							8	1
4					8	5		
	9							7
					5		6	
						3		

Puzzle #34

HARD

9				4			7	
		5			3			
	7		1		9			
			7			5		9
	8			3			6	
			9	6	2	7		
		2		5				
	4				1	8		
			6			2		5

Puzzle #35

HARD

		8					2	
	3		6					8
				4				
	4				7		5	
3					5			1
5	7			2			6	
		2	3				8	6
	1				9			3
						9		

Puzzle #36

HARD

			6			3		8
4	2		8					
				4	5			
3					8	1		
7	5		1				6	
1			3		2			
						8		
	9		2					5
				5			9	

Puzzle #37

HARD

	8	1	9		3			
5				2		8		
		9					6	4
						5		
7	3							
	2	5		7			9	
			6			1		5
				9	4			6
			8					

Puzzle #38

HARD

2				4		7	3	
	5						6	9
	4		5					
5					1	9	4	7
7					6			
	9	1						
	6		3					
	7		9		2			6
		3						8

Puzzle #39

HARD

9			5			2		6
		2	7		4			
1		9						
	7						8	
5				8			6	9
	4		8	2		5		1
				4	1			
	9				3			

Puzzle #40

HARD

	2		3					
					7			1
					8	3	6	
9			2		6	8		
	5					9		
8		4	1				3	
					4	7		
		2	6					
	6	1		7		4		

Puzzle #41

HARD

2		8					4	
				9	2		7	
	1	4						
	9		3			5		
	8	5		7			6	
		3			4			
1					7			3
	3			1			9	6

Puzzle #42

HARD

4		3	2					
	5				8			
8	6		1		5		4	
				8	1			9
			3				1	
	4	7						
		5						
					9	2		
2	3					5	8	

Puzzle #43

HARD

	9			5				
			2			6		
	8						1	
7				6		2		4
8	6		1			7		
							9	
								8
2	5				6			3
			9	4				

Puzzle #44

HARD

						5	8	
							4	
7		6						2
	9				4			8
	1		3		8		6	
				6		3		
9		7			6		1	
5			1			7		4
1	8			3				

Puzzle #45

HARD

		6	8				2	
					4			6
4				3		1		
8			5		6			4
	9					7		
				8			9	2
							3	
5	2			6				
1			4				5	

Puzzle #46

HARD

	5				8		1	
	2			9		4		
		7		6	3			
4						7		2
1		9	5					
3	8							
				1		6		
	6	3				9	7	

Puzzle #47

HARD

1		4		3		8		5
	2			6		1		
7								
8	6		5		3		4	
				9		5		6
		1	7			4	3	
		9			1			
6								

Puzzle #48

HARD

	1	3				5		
		4						9
8					2		4	
	9						7	
	6							5
			5	8		9	6	
			3		1			2
				5		1	9	
7								8

Puzzle #49

HARD

	7			5				
1							6	9
		9	7		3	4		
2			6					
3				2			8	
	8	4						6
					1			8
	2	8					9	
			4		7			5

Puzzle #50

HARD

					4	5		
8		6						4
			1	5				
9					1	2		
7			5					
6	4							7
	3					1		9
					2	8		
2				7				

Puzzle #51

HARD

2										6
				1	2	5				9
	3			6						
	2	9								
7		5				3				
					5			8	7	
						7				8
6		7							9	1
								3		

Puzzle #52

HARD

9		8		1				
	5	6	4					
7		2			3			8
		1		6				
								1
5					9	7		
		5			2		8	
	1		3	8			7	
		9				6		

Puzzle #53

HARD

7	3		4				6	
	5			2			8	4
		3		7	4	1		
9		5						
6					3		7	
			2					1
2					7		4	
	6			5				

Puzzle #54

HARD

			1		6	3		5
	4						9	
2			9			8		6
	9		2					
7				3	1			
		2	6	4				
6								
	5						2	1
						7	8	

Puzzle #55

HARD

2	3					7		
					8			
	9						4	2
		6				3	5	
7			3					
				2	5	6		
					9	5		6
	1		7					
3		4	6					

Puzzle #56

HARD

			5					6
					6	1	7	
8		6		9				
			3					
5	7			2				3
		3		6	8			
					9			2
		8		3		4		
	4		8				1	

Puzzle #57

HARD

		3	6			9		
5		2		9				
					3			
		4		2	7		6	
3	5		9				7	
		9	8					3
4					8	6		
	2		7			4		
8			2					

Puzzle #58

HARD

	4			3			6	
			2			3		
	5			1			8	
3		1		6				7
6	9							
							4	3
	6		5			2		9
			1			4		
			4	8				

Puzzle #59

HARD

	4			9	3			
		9				7		
	2	1	8			6	4	
	6							
			7			5		3
9			3		2	1		
			2					1
				3				7
5		6	9					2

Puzzle #60

HARD

	1	9			3	6	2	
		8			5		4	
			6	9				
4	6		1					5
7				4			1	
		6				2		
	3				7		9	
			8			3		

Puzzle #61

HARD

9		2					3	4
		7			5		9	6
	4	6		2	9			7
	6						4	
			7	8				
							6	
8		5			3			
				5		8		
			1	4				3

Puzzle #62

HARD

			3					
	5			4	9		1	2
			2			4		
		4			1	3		
		7	6	3				8
3	2							
			1					
9	1							6
	6					5	8	

Puzzle #63

HARD

2		7					9	
	3				6			8
	1						4	
	5			9		1		
7		8			4		2	
	2					3		
			6	3				2
			7					
		1		2			7	

Puzzle #64

HARD

		5				1	4	
	2			4			6	9
9				1				7
						5		
			2				1	
	7	1		3				
8								4
			6			7		
		4			5		3	

Puzzle #65

HARD

	3	8						
			7			5	1	
			9	6				
2			8	9				
7			6	2	4		3	
	9	5						6
9	1	2		4	3			7
			2			4		

Puzzle #66

HARD

					4			
		2			5			1
		7		1	6	5	8	
6			8					
			3	7		1		4
		1			9			7
		9	5	4	8		1	
			7			9		
				9	1			

Puzzle #67

HARD

		2						5
	1			6	7			
		6		2		4		
		5	7		3	6		
9								
						2		7
				8				
6			1				9	
3	8		5					4

Puzzle #68

HARD

							1	
	1				6			5
9		4	2		3		
3		8	5		1		
8				9	5		4
							8
	1	2	6	8			
7		3					
	5	8	3		4		

Puzzle #69

HARD

| | 1 | | | 6 | | | | | |
| | 5 | | | | | | | 9 | |
				4	2	1	8		
				3		2			
3					8			5	
	4	9				7			
8				6	3	5		7	
	2							1	
									8

Puzzle #70

HARD

	9		7	6			3	
						9		1
		2		5			4	
					1			8
		4				3	7	
	2	6						4
	4			3	6			
				2		1		
	5				8		2	

Puzzle #71

HARD

2					9		5	
					5	1		7
		1		8		2		
	6			3				2
3			6	4				
	7							
		3	2			5		4
								8
4		9	3					

Puzzle #72

HARD

							7	
5	1	2				6		
		7	8	1	4			2
3		9			8		6	
1	2			6				5
8							4	
		6	5		7	8		
			2					

Puzzle #73

HARD

	2	3	7		4		6	
		7		1				4
		5			3			
			3	9			4	6
	6				5		2	8
		8						
8			1					2
				3				
		4	2					9

Puzzle #74

HARD

6			7					
				3				9
	9	2	8	6			4	
			4		8			5
	6		9	2				1
	2			5		6		
2							8	
7								
	4	8			3			

Puzzle #75

HARD

	6	9		7	2		4	
			4					7
3								
	3		1					
1				4	9			8
			6					
	2	8				3		
					7		1	
	1				5		9	

Puzzle #76

HARD

		8	9					2
7				1				9
	2					3	5	
4							9	3
2				6			8	
6				5				
		3	7		9			
		5	8		4		6	

Puzzle #77

HARD

		5		2				
					3	9		
			7	8	9			
		4	1					
7	2							
3	5				6	2	7	
	7		8				5	
4		2						1
				6				

Puzzle #78

HARD

			8	9			5	
3								
	8	7		1	3			2
7	9						8	
6				3		1		
2								9
				4				8
					2		7	
	3		1	6			9	

Puzzle #79

HARD

			8	1				3
		3						
					2	1		4
4		6	9		3		7	
		7		5		9		
5	8							6
3					5			7
					4	5		
			8				9	

Puzzle #80

HARD

		6						9
				5				
9			1			3	7	
				9				
	8		2			7		
	5							8
7		5	4			1	6	
		1	9				3	
6				7				

Puzzle #81

HARD

		5			2			
	4	9	1		5			
			9				8	3
				7			3	
1		7		6			5	
						8	2	
3								8
				2		7	1	
4		6						

Puzzle #82

HARD

					1	2	8	3	
	3	7	5				1		6
8		1			7	2		9	
	7	2			6	4			
3	9			8				6	5
	8		4						
7	5		1			6	8		
		8	7				2		
		3		5		9			

Puzzle #83

HARD

1		2	9					
			2				4	
				8				3
	3				1	5		
	7		8			6		
			5					7
	4			1	2			
	5						7	
2			3	6				1

Puzzle #84

HARD

	8	7	5					4
	9			8	1	5		
		2						1
			9					
			8			7		
3				2			4	
9		8						
	5		1		3		2	
							5	3

Puzzle #85

HARD

	6	9			1		4	
5	3				8			2
				7		3		
6						2	9	
			8					
		7		5	3			
	8		4					
2							8	
			3					5

Puzzle #86

HARD

	6		5					7
			4	2				
		1		6				
4	2			5			3	
	7	9				6		
1						8	4	
	4		3				8	
3			7		1	5		

Puzzle #87
HARD

3	6				7	2		1
			8					
8				4				
6						8		
				5	6			2
1	2		9					
	9	5		6	8			
				3			5	
			2			4		

Puzzle #88

HARD

								8
6	3				1	2		
1			8				5	
2	9	7			8			
			7					4
					9	5		
		6		9				
				4	2	3		
	7							

Puzzle #89

HARD

4					7			2
			4			8		
3			6					
6	8							7
		9		1				8
		4					5	
							6	
		7	2	4			9	3
2	6		3	5				

Puzzle #90

HARD

					7			
4		6				2		
3	8	1		6				
		2	6			7	4	
	5							
				4			6	
	1			7				
			1		9	8		
8			4			3	9	

Puzzle #91

HARD

	4					7	2	
		8			9			
7				3		5		4
	7		6	4				
				9	8		7	
			3					
							8	5
3	8				6			
		4	5					

Puzzle #92

HARD

	5	2			8			
3	9		2			6		
1				7	5			
					2	3		
			9	4	7			5
4	1					9		
						1	6	
				6				
				5				9

Puzzle #93

HARD

	6		5			1		
1	3							9
4		2						
		5	2				1	
	4			6	8	2		7
		8	9	5				
6			8	1				
				4			3	

Puzzle #94

HARD

	3			9	7		2	8
9	8				4		7	
			2					
	2	8				3		7
6			3					
					8		4	
			7	1			9	
	4				6			
7		5				1		

Puzzle #95

HARD

2								
4		8	9		2	1		
			3	4		9		
		6	7	2	9			
						4		
				3				5
		9	4	5	6			
8	6	4						2
						3		

Puzzle #96

HARD

		4		5			6	
				9		8	5	
				2				3
		6				1	9	
9					6			
			2	3				
	4	2			7			5
6		1						
8							4	7

Puzzle #97

HARD

		9					6	8
	4				8			7
	5		2			3		
	6				2	1		
			4					
			9				3	5
4			3				7	
	1						2	
	8		5					4

Puzzle #98

HARD

5		8						3
					2		5	
9	3		1				7	
6			2	1		7		
		7		9		5	3	4
					9		6	
1	9			6	4			
3			8					

Puzzle #99

HARD

			2					
	2	5	4			9		
7				5			8	
	7						4	
			7	1				
9		6				1		
		1						3
8				6	4			
	5		3		2	8		

Puzzle #100

HARD

	8		1	2		5		
			3		5		8	
						6		
3		1		9				7
		2	6		8		4	
6								3
4	5				1	7		
			4	7				

Puzzle #101

HARD

		5	8	7				4
4			9					
6	7					8	9	
		8	4			1		
					1			
5				6				2
	3				5		4	
		2				7		
		9						5

Puzzle #102

HARD

7		2		1				
9	1			4				
					8			
			5			1		
	9						7	
6	5				7			8
4			2					
			1			6		
				9	5	3	2	7

Puzzle #103

HARD

					9	5	4	2
7								
	4	2			3			
			9					
				1			8	3
	8	4	6				1	
		1						8
6					5	7		
2	5		1					

Puzzle #104

HARD

		1	4	9			5	
7		8						3
	5						1	
	9				2	6		
8		7	5					
6					1	8		9
			6	7				
					8	9		
								2

Puzzle #105

HARD

			7		2	1	8	
	6		5					4
	4							
		7	3			5		9
		6				4		
							1	3
					8		2	
8			1		3	9		7
				9		8		

Puzzle #106

HARD

		7					6	
	5		7		1			
	8			2		5		3
					3		8	
		9			7		2	
						4		5
	2	5	9	1	8			
1		6		5				
			6					

Puzzle #107

HARD

				7	6			
8	4		5				1	
			2					5
			6	8				2
	6					9		
					7	5		
	3					1		9
	5	7	9				4	
				2	1			

Puzzle #108

HARD

5		9		4			3	
	6	1				9	7		
	8			7		6			
					3				
		4					1		
		6				5			4
				6				1	
1								2	6
		9				7	3		

Puzzle #109

HARD

5			1			2		
	9			8			5	7
					3			
				2		6		
		3	6			1	7	
			4	7				
3		6			2			
	4		5					
1		5						8

Puzzle #110

HARD

5	6							
2	7					1	8	
					4			7
			9					3
	8				2		5	
				5		9		
		6	7	9		2		
		9	2	4	5	3	7	
					1			

Puzzle #111

HARD

	7							2
4				7			9	1
5			1					
	8	5			1	2		6
				9		5		
3				4				
		4						
	3		8			9		
				6			8	7

Puzzle #112

HARD

					7			
			6					
			3	1		5	6	
5		1						9
	6	9		7		8		
7								
	8	6		9		1		5
						3	4	
		3			2		8	6

Puzzle #113

HARD

		8			5			
		4	7				6	
			6			4		
7						3	8	
1			4		9			
				6				1
							3	
	8				2		7	5
6	2						9	

Puzzle #114

HARD

6			9		4	3		
	3						5	
9		5			1			4
		2						
4	7						9	
					6	2		1
		6		9				
3						9		2
		1			5		7	

Puzzle #115

HARD

	3			1	7			5
	6					7		
		5	9					
5			6			8	4	
	4	1						
7			1				3	2
		8		5		9		
6							1	
2								

Puzzle #116

HARD

1			5	8	2			
	2	3	1					
			4			5		6
		8		2		7	4	
				6				9
	3			9				
6							8	
					3		7	1

Puzzle #117

HARD

6			5					
	9		1					7
					4	5		8
9				7				
7						2		5
		5	8					
			6	5			2	
			2	3		4		1
			7				9	

Puzzle #118

HARD

		5						
6	3					9	4	
			6					7
	9						3	8
		1	7					
				6				2
				2	5		8	
9	1							
8				4	9			3

Puzzle #119

HARD

			7					4
3			2		1			
	2			9			8	
6			5					
		5				3		7
				8				
			6			2	4	8
		2		3			5	6
7					4			

Puzzle #120

HARD

	8	9		6				1
			8	1		4		
	3		4				2	
9								
								8
7		6					4	3
			1				7	
						5	3	6
	7				2			

Puzzle #121

HARD

							9	1	
6	7			3				4
	5	4						
	1	8			9	3		
9			8			7		
			1		2			
	8	3						
		1	2				3	
							5	2

Puzzle #122

HARD

9				4				
						9		3
	8		3	1			5	
		7	6	2				
			1			8	9	
						4		
			2	8		1		
3	6							
		2	7	5			4	

Puzzle #123

HARD

1						4				2
				2				4		3
2									6	
		2		3						
9	3							6	8	
		4		8					2	5
				6						
					2	9				
8				5	3					7

Puzzle #124

HARD

	8				4			
			6				1	9
6					1			7
				4		3		
					6	5	7	
					9		4	8
	1			5				
		4	1		3			
7		8				6		

Puzzle #125

HARD

1	4		9	7		8	3	
3	2		6	5				
		6				9		5
		7		3	4	6	5	
								4
	1		5		9	3	7	
		4		9		7	8	1
		8	7					3
	6			8	5	2		

Puzzle #126

HARD

		8					5	
3					1			9
1					9			
	2		9		8			
		7		5		3		1
							6	
9							4	6
	5		4					7
				7				

Puzzle #127

HARD

		3	4	6				9
				7		3		
	6		2					
9						5		
				8				1
	2						6	
		5	7		1			
	9					2	4	
4								8

Puzzle #128

HARD

			7				6	
1		6			8			9
8				5				
	2		9		4			
		1			2			
		7		9		6	5	
	5		2			7		1
			3				9	8

Puzzle #129

HARD

					9	2		4
	3		1		2			
		9		7				5
		1						2
			2	3	7	6		
				9			8	
2		4				5		
			7	6				
	9		8				4	6

Puzzle #130

HARD

			6		5			
8	2		9					
	4		7				3	5
	1					9		
		6						
3				2			6	7
		3	5					
7		4	3		6		2	
	8							

Puzzle #131

HARD

2							8		6		
				9	4					
5						3				
8				1	7					
					9				5	
7	5	4		2						1
										7
		2				9			1	
					1			3	8	

Puzzle #132

HARD

		3						
8	2			5				
4			1	9				8
3			5		2	7		
				4				2
		4	6				1	
	4							
			9	8		5	3	4
		6						

Puzzle #133

HARD

8	7	6				9		
	9		6	1		2		
1							3	
6		5	8					
			4					1
				2				
					4			
		2		9	7	3	6	
				3				2

Puzzle #134

HARD

	7			4				
	3				7	2	9	
		6				4		3
4					1			
	9			5		7		
		3		9	8			
2		1						
						5		8
	6	9			2		1	

Puzzle #135

HARD

					2	1		
		2	3		5			6
6				8				
								7
3		1	8			9	5	
	5			2		8		
7	4	8						
1					9	4		
9							1	

Puzzle #136

HARD

			7	2				
	2				4	8		
1					6			
		1				3		
				7			6	
	9		5			1	8	
4								7
		9		6	5			
3	8							

Puzzle #137

HARD

		2	7					9
	1			4				2
			5	3				
							5	
2	9					6		
	7	3	8	1				
						2	9	
	4	1	3					
6						8		

Puzzle #138

HARD

				4		5	7	2
	4		9					8
			1					
6						3	5	
3					6			1
		8						
			6	5				
	5						2	
1			4	9	3	7		

Puzzle #139

HARD

5		9					2	
		1		4	8			
							3	
2				1	4			9
	5							
			6			3		
			3	5		6		
3	1			2		8		
7		5			9			

Puzzle #140

HARD

		6	2	9			8
	9	3	6	7			5
			8				
			6			1	2
5		7					
	1	7	9				
			4		7	1	
				8			
	9	1		2			

Puzzle #141

HARD

	3							5
4					6		3	9
			7					
8				9			1	
					2	5		
	2	1			7			
9		8						
			6	1			8	
		6	2	4				

Puzzle #142

HARD

	4		9			2		
				3				7
6	7				1	8	3	
	1	4		2				
								4
	6	5				9	2	
3			4			6		8
	8		6				5	
			7			3		

Puzzle #143

HARD

		6			3			
				8	9			
7			2					
			8	1			6	
6					4	5	7	
8				7	5			9
		5			6		9	
	7			4		1		
		3					5	

Puzzle #144

HARD

	3			6					
---	---	---		---	---	---	---	---	---
6		8		7					2	
						5				
	7		4					
1	5	2					6		
			2	3				1	
				2		3			
							7		
	1		3		7			9

Puzzle #145

HARD

7			2				1	
1		3						4
	9	6			4		7	
			7		6			
5		4	1				9	
		1			2			
					8			9
			3					
2						6		

Puzzle #146

HARD

7								
		5			4			
		4	7			1	8	
1					8	6	2	
				5				9
	5		3			4	1	
	1			7			3	
	7		8					6
6					2			

Puzzle #147

HARD

2						7		
	3			6		4		
		5			2		1	6
			2		9	3	6	
				5	8			9
		1	4	7				
6								7
	4	3				9		5

Puzzle #148

HARD

9	7				6		5	
	2					6		3
	4			1			2	
			9					8
		6	4			7		
						4		
			5					
5				4				9
		2			1		6	

Puzzle #149

HARD

		1			2			3
		3		5		9	7	
							4	
								7
4			5		8		1	
2		8					6	9
	9				6			
3	1							
		6	9					8

Puzzle #150

HARD

	4			9	3	8		
5				8				
			2		1			7
						4		2
	8							
	9	2					1	
				5		7		
		3	8					1
			6			5		8

Puzzle #151

HARD

6							7	1
	8				1			
				9		6		
4		7	1				8	
8	5		6	2				3
					3	4		
1	3							
		2	4			9		

Puzzle #152

HARD

		7					6	
2							3	
	6							8
5			6					
8		3			4			
	1			9			5	
3			8	4				9
		4		5	2			7
			3				2	

Puzzle #153

HARD

		9			5		2	
		4			6			
	3		4			7		9
	2							
				1			4	
5		3			2			
8			7		1			
				3			6	
	6		5					2

Puzzle #154

HARD

		6						
		5		1	2			4
7							1	6
					5	9	4	
4		3	9			6		
9						7		2
					1		2	
		7			8			
			3	9		8		

Puzzle #155

HARD

								9
			4	7		3		
7							2	
8					3	2		
								8
2				1		4		6
4					8	7		
		7		9				2
	9		1	3				

Puzzle #156

HARD

				3	6	8		6
				3	6	8		
			1			7	9	
	2	6				9		
9				8	5		4	
			6		4			
6								5
	5	8						1
	3		4					

Puzzle #157

HARD

	2				8		9	
		4		3				
6						2		
		3		7				6
	1			8			5	
		6						
3						8	2	
	4						6	
	5		2	9				7

Puzzle #158

HARD

2	4					7		
		8		4				
			1		7		3	
	2		6					
3		7		8	2			5
					5	6		
	3			7		2		
			9					8
		5					9	

Puzzle #159

HARD

9			5					
						6	4	
		8					3	
	6			1				
				7		2	5	
		5	9				8	
					1			9
3		2						
	4	7		2				

Puzzle #160

HARD

2	9							
		7	8					5
				3			2	
				5			4	
			6			2	8	3
	8	6			4			
		4		8			9	
1					7	6		4
						1		

Puzzle #161

HARD

		8		4			1	
3		6			7			
2					9		3	
		5	2		3		7	
					4			2
9								
7					2	5		
								3
6	1			5				

Puzzle #162

HARD

5							9	
	3				7	2		
	8			2				4
6	4				3			
			7	1		4		
	2				8	6		
	5					3		
			9	7				
		4			2	7		

Puzzle #163

HARD

				4	7	2		
		1						4
7	6				5	3		
8	5		7		3		2	
			5				6	
					8			
	8				4			
				1		7		
		7	8		6			3

Puzzle #164

HARD

1							9	
5								6
	8				3	7		5
	2		4				7	
				1	9	3		
					8	6		
		6	9			2		
9	3				6	1	4	
				3	7			

Puzzle #165

HARD

			4	9				
	3			2		4		9
	4				1			
6						8	2	
		5					1	
4		7	5					
5			1	6		9		
		3	2	7				
	9				3			

Puzzle #166

HARD

					6			
		2				4		9
	7							1
4			9		1	8		
	8			5				
		5			3			2
		3		9	8			
		4	6	3		7		
		1	5					

Puzzle #167

HARD

			3					4
			9	8	7		5	
	1				5			
7	4			1		8		
				7				2
			6	9			3	1
	9	1						5
2							8	
4	3							

Puzzle #168

HARD

	4	6		7			9	3
	9							
1		3					7	
			3		8	5		
7				6				
5		1	4			6	3	
				1	2		6	
					9		2	
			8					

Puzzle #169

HARD

						5	4	
		1			9		8	
	9		7					
4			7	5				
		2					7	4
				6				
	3		8			9		1
		5	9				2	8
	1		3					

Puzzle #170

HARD

					6			9
	8					7		1
		5	3			4		
9	2							
	6				4		2	
		3	9				8	
						3		
			2	1		8	7	
	4	7	5		3			

Puzzle #171

HARD

		6		3		5		7
					8	1		3
	6		3					2
4					1		5	8
	8			7	6			
					7		1	
5							2	
8	4		2					

Puzzle #172

HARD

		5						
						2	7	
	8	2					1	9
				9			2	
	3	7	1					
		1						4
	5			4		9	8	
3					2			7
			7		9		4	

Puzzle #173

HARD

1		6	2				9	
	7			6				3
	4							
					4			
8				5	9	3		1
					1			
		9					6	
	5	8	2					
	1		3	4				2

Puzzle #174

HARD

			5					7
4		5		9				
		8						
7	3			2				
			1				9	6
					8			5
		9		8		7	1	
6	7		9				4	
5					2			3

Puzzle #175

HARD

	5						2	7
					3		9	
2					1			
	3					1		
		9		1			8	
	7		9					5
					6			
		8						6
5	1			8	7			3

Puzzle #176

HARD

	6	8					9	
				4				5
	9		3		7			
	5				9	7		
7	3					2		
		9				8	1	
					5			
					6		3	
				8	1			

Puzzle #177

HARD

		6			8		9	
4	5	8		1			6	
			7		1			
9								
	8		6					5
7					4			
6			4					
	3					8	1	
		9	7					3

Puzzle #178

HARD

	2				9		6	
5	7		6	3		4		
							8	
						3		
6	3		1		5			4
	1			2		6		
	8		7					
					4		3	
7		5			6	9		

Puzzle #179

HARD

				3				
			2				9	
5	4		7					3
	2					4		
		6		4			2	
		8	3	1				
	7	2	9					
				6				
					8	6		

Puzzle #180

HARD

		1		8				3
	6			1		8		5
				4		1		
3			6					
		6		9			3	8
		7			3		9	
					5			6
8	3				2			
				3	4			2

Puzzle #181

HARD

2								1
		7			6	3		
	8		2		7		5	
8	5				3			
		4		9				
		9			8	7		
		2		4				
								3
5	6						1	9

Puzzle #182

HARD

	9					3		7
1	4			3			9	
		2	4					
					1		6	9
				7	6		1	
5			2					
			9				2	
7				1		6		5
							7	

Puzzle #183

HARD

				8	9	5		
			3					1
	5							7
			9		1	2		
5		3		4		8		
			2					3
7	8						2	
	4		7					
6						9		

Puzzle #184

HARD

							9		6
	7		4					8	
8		5			2				
	1			5				9	
							7		
7				1		5			2
2			7						4
6			2						
					3	1			9

Puzzle #185

HARD

	4	5		1	9			
6								3
	3		4					
			2		5			
8					3	7	2	
	9						5	
2		1					8	
	7		6			3		
								7

Puzzle #186

HARD

				5	7			9
	2	7				8	4	
8					3			
		1						8
						4	7	
		8	4	3		5		
	1						3	2
9		4	1					
							5	

Puzzle #187

HARD

	8				1			
					2		6	4
	5	4						
	3		8					
		9	5				1	
			3	7		5		
1			7		5			3
2				9			4	
	7							

Puzzle #188

HARD

8			5		4			
	6		5	1	8			
		7	3					
		2	4					
							5	
	3		7				6	1
			2	3		7		
					1			5
1	4					2		

Puzzle #189

HARD

		1				9		
	3		5	8				
	7				3			
			1	7			3	
6	4							8
						6		
						8		
	5		4		2		6	
2		9					4	1

Puzzle #190

HARD

						6	1	2
9			5			3		
	4				2		5	
8							2	
5				8				
			9					3
6				1			8	
		4					7	
7		5	4			9		

Puzzle #191

HARD

		4					6	
6			2					
	9				3	8		4
4	3	2			1			
	6		4					
				3			5	
	4	9				5		
8			5				1	2
				8				7

Puzzle #192

HARD

				2				
					1			5
			4			8		9
2		8						
			1					6
5			9			1	4	2
		7	8		9	3		
		2		4				
		5					6	

Puzzle #193

HARD

	4				1		6	
	1			3		5		7
		6					3	
7	2		5					
			7			1	8	
			9			3		
		2			4			
4	9							8
					2	4		

Puzzle #194

HARD

		8						
	1							2
	7		5	1				
		6			2			1
		1	7			3		
4	9				1			
				8		2	1	4
7								6
				3	4		7	

Puzzle #195

HARD

			9	6				
	3						5	4
						7		
8		5		4				
	1				7	8		
3				9		4		
1	6			2	4			
			8					
	7	4				1		

Puzzle #196

HARD

				6			7	
		5		9	7	4		
3						1		
				1			8	
	6							7
				8				2
					3			
8	1			4	9			
4	9		5			2		8

Puzzle #197
HARD

1			3	7				
7		6				4		
5	2		4					1
	1		2			7	9	
				5				
	4		3					2
			9					
				2	3	5		
			7	8	5	1	2	

Puzzle #198

HARD

	1				9	5		3
		9		6			2	
6					7	9		
			7			6		8
			2				7	5
		3	8		5			1
1						4		
		8			1			

Puzzle #199

HARD

	4			9				
	9						7	
5	6		8		2	1		
			2	4			9	
				6				
1					5	2		
	5							
				3			8	
			7			9	6	3

Puzzle #200

HARD

Puzzle # 1

3	5	8	2	6	1	7	9	4
2	1	4	7	9	5	8	6	3
6	7	9	4	3	8	2	5	1
7	8	3	6	1	9	4	2	5
4	6	1	5	2	7	9	3	8
5	9	2	8	4	3	6	1	7
8	2	7	3	5	6	1	4	9
9	4	5	1	8	2	3	7	6
1	3	6	9	7	4	5	8	2

Puzzle # 2

5	2	6	8	9	7	1	4	3
3	7	9	6	4	1	5	2	8
1	8	4	3	5	2	6	9	7
9	4	3	7	6	8	2	5	1
2	5	8	9	1	4	7	3	6
6	1	7	2	3	5	9	8	4
4	6	5	1	2	3	8	7	9
8	9	2	4	7	6	3	1	5
7	3	1	5	8	9	4	6	2

Puzzle # 3

3	5	9	8	1	2	7	4	6
7	8	2	4	5	6	3	1	9
6	4	1	3	7	9	2	5	8
4	3	7	1	9	8	5	6	2
1	6	8	7	2	5	9	3	4
9	2	5	6	3	4	1	8	7
5	1	6	2	4	7	8	9	3
8	7	3	9	6	1	4	2	5
2	9	4	5	8	3	6	7	1

Puzzle # 4

1	7	6	5	3	4	8	9	2
4	8	2	6	9	1	3	7	5
5	9	3	7	8	2	4	1	6
6	2	7	3	1	9	5	8	4
3	1	8	4	2	5	9	6	7
9	4	5	8	7	6	1	2	3
7	5	9	2	4	8	6	3	1
8	3	4	1	6	7	2	5	9
2	6	1	9	5	3	7	4	8

Puzzle # 5

5	9	7	1	3	2	6	8	4
6	4	1	7	8	5	3	2	9
2	3	8	9	4	6	5	1	7
7	5	4	3	6	1	8	9	2
1	6	2	8	7	9	4	3	5
9	8	3	5	2	4	7	6	1
3	1	5	6	9	7	2	4	8
8	2	9	4	5	3	1	7	6
4	7	6	2	1	8	9	5	3

Puzzle # 6

8	4	2	3	6	7	9	1	5
9	6	3	4	1	5	8	2	7
7	1	5	8	9	2	4	6	3
1	3	8	7	5	6	2	4	9
2	5	6	9	8	4	7	3	1
4	7	9	2	3	1	5	8	6
6	8	1	5	2	9	3	7	4
3	9	7	6	4	8	1	5	2
5	2	4	1	7	3	6	9	8

Puzzle # 7

9	1	4	2	8	5	6	3	7
8	7	2	4	3	6	5	9	1
3	6	5	9	1	7	4	8	2
1	5	8	6	7	2	9	4	3
6	4	3	1	9	8	7	2	5
7	2	9	5	4	3	1	6	8
4	8	1	3	5	9	2	7	6
5	3	6	7	2	4	8	1	9
2	9	7	8	6	1	3	5	4

Puzzle # 8

6	5	7	1	3	8	4	2	9
2	3	1	9	6	4	8	7	5
4	9	8	7	5	2	1	3	6
7	1	5	2	8	6	3	9	4
8	2	4	3	9	7	6	5	1
9	6	3	4	1	5	7	8	2
3	7	6	5	4	9	2	1	8
5	8	2	6	7	1	9	4	3
1	4	9	8	2	3	5	6	7

Puzzle # 9

3	6	7	5	2	9	1	4	8
5	2	9	8	1	4	3	7	6
4	1	8	6	3	7	2	9	5
9	3	6	7	8	1	5	2	4
7	5	4	2	6	3	8	1	9
1	8	2	4	9	5	6	3	7
6	4	1	3	7	8	9	5	2
8	7	3	9	5	2	4	6	1
2	9	5	1	4	6	7	8	3

Puzzle # 10

1	6	9	8	2	3	5	4	7
3	5	8	4	7	6	2	9	1
2	7	4	1	9	5	8	6	3
6	2	1	3	8	9	4	7	5
5	4	3	7	6	1	9	2	8
9	8	7	2	5	4	3	1	6
8	9	5	6	4	7	1	3	2
7	3	2	9	1	8	6	5	4
4	1	6	5	3	2	7	8	9

Puzzle # 11

4	5	6	1	2	7	9	3	8
1	3	7	8	9	6	4	2	5
2	8	9	4	5	3	7	1	6
6	2	3	9	7	8	5	4	1
7	9	1	5	4	2	8	6	3
5	4	8	3	6	1	2	7	9
9	7	2	6	1	5	3	8	4
3	6	5	7	8	4	1	9	2
8	1	4	2	3	9	6	5	7

Puzzle # 12

2	6	4	9	7	3	1	8	5
9	8	7	1	5	4	2	3	6
3	5	1	6	8	2	4	9	7
8	9	2	3	6	7	5	1	4
7	4	5	2	9	1	3	6	8
6	1	3	8	4	5	9	7	2
4	3	8	5	1	6	7	2	9
1	7	6	4	2	9	8	5	3
5	2	9	7	3	8	6	4	1

Puzzle # 13

5	2	9	8	1	4	3	6	7
8	1	3	2	6	7	5	9	4
7	6	4	5	9	3	8	2	1
1	9	7	3	4	5	2	8	6
3	4	2	6	7	8	9	1	5
6	8	5	1	2	9	7	4	3
9	7	8	4	5	1	6	3	2
2	3	1	7	8	6	4	5	9
4	5	6	9	3	2	1	7	8

Puzzle # 14

7	9	1	3	4	5	6	8	2
8	5	4	2	9	6	1	7	3
3	2	6	1	7	8	5	4	9
4	3	8	6	5	1	9	2	7
5	1	9	8	2	7	3	6	4
6	7	2	4	3	9	8	5	1
9	6	7	5	1	4	2	3	8
2	4	5	9	8	3	7	1	6
1	8	3	7	6	2	4	9	5

Puzzle # 15

9	4	6	7	3	2	8	5	1
8	3	2	6	1	5	9	4	7
1	7	5	8	4	9	2	6	3
4	9	3	5	6	1	7	8	2
2	8	1	3	7	4	6	9	5
5	6	7	2	9	8	1	3	4
3	1	9	4	8	7	5	2	6
7	5	4	9	2	6	3	1	8
6	2	8	1	5	3	4	7	9

Puzzle # 16

7	2	9	1	5	4	6	8	3
4	3	6	7	8	2	5	1	9
1	8	5	6	9	3	4	7	2
9	7	2	5	3	6	8	4	1
8	1	4	9	2	7	3	6	5
5	6	3	8	4	1	2	9	7
2	5	7	4	6	9	1	3	8
6	9	8	3	1	5	7	2	4
3	4	1	2	7	8	9	5	6

Puzzle # 17

7	2	5	9	1	6	3	4	8
4	9	6	2	3	8	7	5	1
8	1	3	4	7	5	9	6	2
1	6	2	3	4	7	8	9	5
5	3	4	8	6	9	2	1	7
9	8	7	5	2	1	4	3	6
2	7	9	6	5	3	1	8	4
6	4	8	1	9	2	5	7	3
3	5	1	7	8	4	6	2	9

Puzzle # 18

1	8	7	3	9	2	5	6	4
5	2	9	8	4	6	7	1	3
6	3	4	1	5	7	9	8	2
4	5	6	2	8	3	1	9	7
8	9	1	4	7	5	2	3	6
3	7	2	9	6	1	8	4	5
7	1	5	6	3	9	4	2	8
9	4	3	5	2	8	6	7	1
2	6	8	7	1	4	3	5	9

Puzzle # 19

8	7	4	9	2	5	3	6	1
9	2	1	6	8	3	4	7	5
6	5	3	1	4	7	2	9	8
4	8	5	3	9	6	1	2	7
2	9	6	7	1	4	5	8	3
1	3	7	2	5	8	9	4	6
5	1	8	4	7	2	6	3	9
3	4	9	8	6	1	7	5	2
7	6	2	5	3	9	8	1	4

Puzzle # 20

1	9	3	7	6	4	5	8	2
5	4	6	2	8	9	1	7	3
2	8	7	5	3	1	9	4	6
7	6	1	9	4	8	2	3	5
9	5	8	3	2	7	6	1	4
4	3	2	1	5	6	8	9	7
3	1	9	6	7	5	4	2	8
8	2	5	4	1	3	7	6	9
6	7	4	8	9	2	3	5	1

Puzzle # 21

9	4	5	6	2	7	3	8	1
7	6	2	3	8	1	4	5	9
3	8	1	5	4	9	6	2	7
4	9	8	2	6	5	1	7	3
2	1	7	9	3	4	8	6	5
6	5	3	7	1	8	2	9	4
5	2	6	1	7	3	9	4	8
1	7	4	8	9	2	5	3	6
8	3	9	4	5	6	7	1	2

Puzzle # 22

5	7	2	1	3	6	4	8	9
1	8	6	4	9	5	7	3	2
3	4	9	8	2	7	5	1	6
4	9	7	5	1	3	6	2	8
2	1	5	6	7	8	9	4	3
6	3	8	2	4	9	1	7	5
8	2	1	9	5	4	3	6	7
7	5	4	3	6	2	8	9	1
9	6	3	7	8	1	2	5	4

Puzzle # 23

1	7	8	2	5	4	3	9	6
4	2	3	9	8	6	1	7	5
5	6	9	3	1	7	2	8	4
7	3	1	4	2	8	6	5	9
6	4	2	5	9	1	8	3	7
8	9	5	7	6	3	4	1	2
2	8	7	6	3	5	9	4	1
3	5	6	1	4	9	7	2	8
9	1	4	8	7	2	5	6	3

Puzzle # 24

6	1	3	2	8	9	4	7	5
5	9	4	7	6	3	1	2	8
2	7	8	4	5	1	6	9	3
7	4	2	3	1	6	5	8	9
1	8	5	9	2	4	7	3	6
9	3	6	8	7	5	2	4	1
8	6	9	5	4	2	3	1	7
3	2	1	6	9	7	8	5	4
4	5	7	1	3	8	9	6	2

Puzzle # 25

2	3	4	8	5	6	9	7	1
6	9	1	3	7	2	5	8	4
7	8	5	9	4	1	6	2	3
1	2	3	7	6	5	4	9	8
9	4	8	1	2	3	7	5	6
5	6	7	4	9	8	3	1	2
3	1	9	6	8	7	2	4	5
4	5	6	2	1	9	8	3	7
8	7	2	5	3	4	1	6	9

Puzzle # 26

5	4	3	6	2	9	8	7	1
7	1	2	3	5	8	9	6	4
8	9	6	4	7	1	2	5	3
3	8	4	5	9	2	6	1	7
2	7	9	1	4	6	3	8	5
1	6	5	7	8	3	4	2	9
6	5	8	9	1	4	7	3	2
9	2	7	8	3	5	1	4	6
4	3	1	2	6	7	5	9	8

Puzzle # 27

7	3	8	4	1	5	9	6	2
4	6	2	8	9	7	5	3	1
1	9	5	2	3	6	8	4	7
3	2	6	1	7	8	4	9	5
9	1	4	6	5	3	2	7	8
5	8	7	9	2	4	3	1	6
2	4	1	5	6	9	7	8	3
6	7	9	3	8	2	1	5	4
8	5	3	7	4	1	6	2	9

Puzzle # 28

3	6	8	9	2	5	1	7	4
4	5	2	7	3	1	6	8	9
7	9	1	8	6	4	3	5	2
1	4	6	5	9	8	2	3	7
9	2	7	6	4	3	8	1	5
5	8	3	1	7	2	4	9	6
6	7	4	3	1	9	5	2	8
8	1	9	2	5	6	7	4	3
2	3	5	4	8	7	9	6	1

Puzzle # 29

7	3	2	6	1	8	9	5	4
5	6	8	4	2	9	7	1	3
4	9	1	7	5	3	6	8	2
1	4	6	9	3	5	2	7	8
3	8	7	2	4	1	5	6	9
2	5	9	8	6	7	4	3	1
8	2	5	3	9	6	1	4	7
6	7	4	1	8	2	3	9	5
9	1	3	5	7	4	8	2	6

Puzzle # 30

9	2	1	6	3	5	4	8	7
7	8	5	9	1	4	3	2	6
6	3	4	7	2	8	1	5	9
2	9	6	4	8	7	5	3	1
5	4	3	1	6	9	8	7	2
1	7	8	2	5	3	9	6	4
3	1	9	8	7	2	6	4	5
8	6	7	5	4	1	2	9	3
4	5	2	3	9	6	7	1	8

Puzzle # 31

4	2	6	1	5	9	8	3	7
3	8	7	6	4	2	5	1	9
5	9	1	3	8	7	6	2	4
9	7	4	5	1	3	2	8	6
2	6	5	7	9	8	3	4	1
8	1	3	4	2	6	7	9	5
7	3	9	2	6	4	1	5	8
6	5	8	9	3	1	4	7	2
1	4	2	8	7	5	9	6	3

Puzzle # 32

6	4	3	8	9	1	2	5	7
2	9	5	4	3	7	8	1	6
1	7	8	5	6	2	9	4	3
8	2	1	7	5	9	6	3	4
4	6	9	1	8	3	5	7	2
3	5	7	6	2	4	1	9	8
9	8	2	3	7	5	4	6	1
7	1	6	9	4	8	3	2	5
5	3	4	2	1	6	7	8	9

Puzzle # 33

9	8	3	1	2	4	6	7	5
2	4	6	5	7	9	8	1	3
1	7	5	6	8	3	4	9	2
8	5	1	2	3	6	7	4	9
6	3	9	4	5	7	2	8	1
4	2	7	9	1	8	5	3	6
3	9	4	8	6	2	1	5	7
7	1	2	3	4	5	9	6	8
5	6	8	7	9	1	3	2	4

Puzzle # 34

9	2	8	5	4	6	3	7	1
6	1	5	8	7	3	9	2	4
3	7	4	1	2	9	6	5	8
2	6	3	7	1	8	5	4	9
7	8	9	4	3	5	1	6	2
4	5	1	9	6	2	7	8	3
8	9	2	3	5	7	4	1	6
5	4	6	2	9	1	8	3	7
1	3	7	6	8	4	2	9	5

Puzzle # 35

1	6	8	7	9	3	4	2	5
7	3	4	6	5	2	1	9	8
2	9	5	8	4	1	6	3	7
8	4	6	1	3	7	2	5	9
3	2	9	4	6	5	8	7	1
5	7	1	9	2	8	3	6	4
9	5	2	3	1	4	7	8	6
6	1	7	2	8	9	5	4	3
4	8	3	5	7	6	9	1	2

Puzzle # 36

9	1	5	6	2	7	3	4	8
4	2	6	8	1	3	9	5	7
8	3	7	9	4	5	6	1	2
3	4	2	5	6	8	1	7	9
7	5	8	1	9	4	2	6	3
1	6	9	3	7	2	5	8	4
5	7	1	4	3	9	8	2	6
6	9	4	2	8	1	7	3	5
2	8	3	7	5	6	4	9	1

Puzzle # 37

6	8	1	9	4	3	2	5	7
5	4	3	7	2	6	8	1	9
2	7	9	1	5	8	3	6	4
9	1	4	3	6	2	5	7	8
7	3	6	5	8	9	4	2	1
8	2	5	4	7	1	6	9	3
4	9	2	6	3	7	1	8	5
1	5	8	2	9	4	7	3	6
3	6	7	8	1	5	9	4	2

Puzzle # 38

2	1	8	6	4	9	7	3	5
3	5	7	2	1	8	4	6	9
6	4	9	5	7	3	8	2	1
5	3	6	8	2	1	9	4	7
7	8	2	4	9	6	1	5	3
4	9	1	7	3	5	6	8	2
1	6	5	3	8	7	2	9	4
8	7	4	9	5	2	3	1	6
9	2	3	1	6	4	5	7	8

Puzzle # 39

9	1	7	5	3	8	2	4	6
4	6	8	2	1	9	3	7	5
3	5	2	7	6	4	9	1	8
1	8	9	3	7	6	4	5	2
2	7	6	4	9	5	1	8	3
5	3	4	1	8	2	7	6	9
6	4	3	8	2	7	5	9	1
8	2	5	9	4	1	6	3	7
7	9	1	6	5	3	8	2	4

Puzzle # 40

4	2	7	3	6	1	5	8	9
6	3	8	9	5	7	2	4	1
1	9	5	4	2	8	3	6	7
9	1	3	2	4	6	8	7	5
2	5	6	7	8	3	9	1	4
8	7	4	1	9	5	6	3	2
3	8	9	5	1	4	7	2	6
7	4	2	6	3	9	1	5	8
5	6	1	8	7	2	4	9	3

Puzzle # 41

2	7	8	5	3	1	6	4	9
3	5	6	4	9	2	1	7	8
9	1	4	7	6	8	2	3	5
7	9	1	3	2	6	5	8	4
4	8	5	1	7	9	3	6	2
6	2	3	8	5	4	9	1	7
1	6	2	9	4	7	8	5	3
5	4	9	6	8	3	7	2	1
8	3	7	2	1	5	4	9	6

Puzzle # 42

4	7	3	2	9	6	1	5	8
9	5	1	7	4	8	3	2	6
8	6	2	1	3	5	9	4	7
3	2	6	5	8	1	4	7	9
5	9	8	3	7	4	6	1	2
1	4	7	9	6	2	8	3	5
6	8	5	4	2	3	7	9	1
7	1	4	8	5	9	2	6	3
2	3	9	6	1	7	5	8	4

Puzzle # 43

3	9	2	6	5	1	8	4	7
1	4	7	2	3	8	6	5	9
5	8	6	4	9	7	3	1	2
7	1	5	3	6	9	2	8	4
8	6	9	1	2	4	7	3	5
4	2	3	7	8	5	1	9	6
9	3	1	5	7	2	4	6	8
2	5	4	8	1	6	9	7	3
6	7	8	9	4	3	5	2	1

Puzzle # 44

3	2	9	6	4	1	5	8	7
8	5	1	2	9	7	6	4	3
7	4	6	8	5	3	1	9	2
6	9	3	5	1	4	2	7	8
2	1	5	3	7	8	4	6	9
4	7	8	9	6	2	3	5	1
9	3	7	4	2	6	8	1	5
5	6	2	1	8	9	7	3	4
1	8	4	7	3	5	9	2	6

Puzzle # 45

7	5	6	8	1	9	4	2	3
2	3	1	7	5	4	9	8	6
4	8	9	6	3	2	1	7	5
8	7	2	5	9	6	3	1	4
3	9	5	2	4	1	7	6	8
6	1	4	3	8	7	5	9	2
9	4	8	1	2	5	6	3	7
5	2	7	9	6	3	8	4	1
1	6	3	4	7	8	2	5	9

Puzzle # 46

7	5	4	2	3	8	6	1	9
6	2	3	1	9	5	4	7	8
8	9	1	7	4	6	3	2	5
4	6	9	8	1	3	7	5	2
1	7	2	9	5	4	8	3	6
3	8	5	6	2	7	9	4	1
9	3	8	5	7	1	2	6	4
5	4	6	3	8	2	1	9	7
2	1	7	4	6	9	5	8	3

Puzzle # 47

1	7	4	9	3	2	8	6	5
9	3	6	1	8	5	7	2	4
5	2	8	4	6	7	1	9	3
7	9	5	6	1	4	3	8	2
8	6	2	5	7	3	9	4	1
4	1	3	2	9	8	5	7	6
2	8	1	7	5	6	4	3	9
3	4	9	8	2	1	6	5	7
6	5	7	3	4	9	2	1	8

Puzzle # 48

9	1	3	7	4	8	5	2	6
6	2	4	1	3	5	7	8	9
8	7	5	9	6	2	3	4	1
5	9	8	6	1	3	2	7	4
3	6	7	4	2	9	8	1	5
1	4	2	5	8	7	9	6	3
4	8	9	3	7	1	6	5	2
2	3	6	8	5	4	1	9	7
7	5	1	2	9	6	4	3	8

Puzzle # 49

4	7	2	9	5	6	8	1	3
1	5	3	8	4	2	7	6	9
8	6	9	7	1	3	4	5	2
2	9	7	6	3	8	5	4	1
3	1	6	5	2	4	9	8	7
5	8	4	1	7	9	2	3	6
6	4	5	2	9	1	3	7	8
7	2	8	3	6	5	1	9	4
9	3	1	4	8	7	6	2	5

Puzzle # 50

1	9	2	6	4	7	5	3	8
8	5	6	2	9	3	7	1	4
3	7	4	1	5	8	6	9	2
9	8	5	7	3	1	2	4	6
7	2	3	5	6	4	9	8	1
6	4	1	8	2	9	3	5	7
5	3	7	4	8	6	1	2	9
4	6	9	3	1	2	8	7	5
2	1	8	9	7	5	4	6	3

Puzzle # 51

2	5	1	3	4	9	7	8	6
8	7	6	1	2	5	4	3	9
9	3	4	6	7	8	2	1	5
4	2	9	7	8	6	1	5	3
7	8	5	2	1	3	9	6	4
1	6	3	9	5	4	8	7	2
3	1	2	5	9	7	6	4	8
6	4	7	8	3	2	5	9	1
5	9	8	4	6	1	3	2	7

Puzzle # 52

9	3	8	2	1	7	4	6	5
1	5	6	4	9	8	3	2	7
7	4	2	6	5	3	9	1	8
4	2	1	7	6	5	8	9	3
6	9	7	8	3	4	2	5	1
5	8	3	1	2	9	7	4	6
3	6	5	9	7	2	1	8	4
2	1	4	3	8	6	5	7	9
8	7	9	5	4	1	6	3	2

Puzzle # 53

7	3	8	4	1	5	9	6	2
1	5	6	3	2	9	7	8	4
4	9	2	7	6	8	5	1	3
8	2	3	6	7	4	1	5	9
9	7	5	1	8	2	4	3	6
6	4	1	5	9	3	2	7	8
5	8	7	2	4	6	3	9	1
2	1	9	8	3	7	6	4	5
3	6	4	9	5	1	8	2	7

Puzzle # 54

9	7	8	1	2	6	3	4	5
1	4	6	3	8	5	2	9	7
2	5	3	9	7	4	8	1	6
8	9	1	2	5	7	4	6	3
7	6	4	8	3	1	9	5	2
5	3	2	6	4	9	1	7	8
6	2	7	4	1	8	5	3	9
4	8	5	7	9	3	6	2	1
3	1	9	5	6	2	7	8	4

Puzzle # 55

2	3	8	5	9	4	7	6	1
4	6	1	2	7	8	9	3	5
5	9	7	1	6	3	8	4	2
9	2	6	8	1	7	3	5	4
7	8	5	3	4	6	1	2	9
1	4	3	9	2	5	6	7	8
8	7	2	4	3	9	5	1	6
6	1	9	7	5	2	4	8	3
3	5	4	6	8	1	2	9	7

Puzzle # 56

7	1	4	5	8	3	9	2	6
9	3	5	2	4	6	1	7	8
8	2	6	1	9	7	5	3	4
6	8	2	3	1	5	7	4	9
5	7	1	9	2	4	8	6	3
4	9	3	7	6	8	2	5	1
1	6	7	4	5	9	3	8	2
2	5	8	6	3	1	4	9	7
3	4	9	8	7	2	6	1	5

Puzzle # 57

7	1	3	6	8	2	9	5	4
5	6	2	4	9	1	3	8	7
9	4	8	5	7	3	2	1	6
1	8	4	3	2	7	5	6	9
3	5	6	9	1	4	8	7	2
2	7	9	8	6	5	1	4	3
4	9	7	1	3	8	6	2	5
6	2	1	7	5	9	4	3	8
8	3	5	2	4	6	7	9	1

Puzzle # 58

8	4	9	7	3	5	1	6	2
1	7	6	2	4	8	3	9	5
2	5	3	6	1	9	7	8	4
3	2	1	8	6	4	9	5	7
6	9	4	3	5	7	8	2	1
7	8	5	9	2	1	6	4	3
4	6	8	5	7	3	2	1	9
5	3	2	1	9	6	4	7	8
9	1	7	4	8	2	5	3	6

Puzzle # 59

8	4	7	6	9	3	2	1	5
6	5	9	4	2	1	7	3	8
3	2	1	8	7	5	6	4	9
7	6	3	1	5	9	8	2	4
2	1	4	7	8	6	5	9	3
9	8	5	3	4	2	1	7	6
4	3	8	2	6	7	9	5	1
1	9	2	5	3	8	4	6	7
5	7	6	9	1	4	3	8	2

Puzzle # 60

5	1	9	4	7	3	6	2	8
6	7	8	2	1	5	9	4	3
2	4	3	6	9	8	5	7	1
4	6	2	1	8	9	7	3	5
7	9	5	3	4	6	8	1	2
3	8	1	7	5	2	4	6	9
1	5	6	9	3	4	2	8	7
8	3	4	5	2	7	1	9	6
9	2	7	8	6	1	3	5	4

Puzzle # 61

9	5	2	8	6	7	1	3	4
3	8	7	4	1	5	2	9	6
1	4	6	3	2	9	5	8	7
7	6	8	5	9	1	3	4	2
4	2	3	7	8	6	9	1	5
5	9	1	2	3	4	7	6	8
8	1	5	6	7	3	4	2	9
6	3	4	9	5	2	8	7	1
2	7	9	1	4	8	6	5	3

Puzzle # 62

2	4	6	3	1	5	8	7	9
8	5	3	7	4	9	6	1	2
1	7	9	2	6	8	4	5	3
6	8	4	5	9	1	3	2	7
5	9	7	6	3	2	1	4	8
3	2	1	4	8	7	9	6	5
7	3	8	1	5	6	2	9	4
9	1	5	8	2	4	7	3	6
4	6	2	9	7	3	5	8	1

Puzzle # 63

2	8	7	4	5	3	6	9	1
9	3	4	1	7	6	2	5	8
5	1	6	9	8	2	7	4	3
4	5	3	2	9	8	1	6	7
7	6	8	3	1	4	5	2	9
1	2	9	5	6	7	3	8	4
8	7	5	6	3	9	4	1	2
6	9	2	7	4	1	8	3	5
3	4	1	8	2	5	9	7	6

Puzzle # 64

3	8	5	7	6	9	1	4	2
1	2	7	5	4	8	3	6	9
9	4	6	3	1	2	8	5	7
4	3	2	9	8	1	5	7	6
6	9	8	2	5	7	4	1	3
5	7	1	4	3	6	2	9	8
8	5	9	1	7	3	6	2	4
2	1	3	6	9	4	7	8	5
7	6	4	8	2	5	9	3	1

Puzzle # 65

1	3	8	4	5	2	7	6	9
6	4	9	7	3	8	5	1	2
5	2	7	9	6	1	3	4	8
2	6	3	8	9	5	1	7	4
7	8	1	6	2	4	9	3	5
4	9	5	3	1	7	8	2	6
9	1	2	5	4	3	6	8	7
3	7	6	2	8	9	4	5	1
8	5	4	1	7	6	2	9	3

Puzzle # 66

5	1	3	8	2	4	6	7	9
6	8	2	9	7	5	4	3	1
4	9	7	3	1	6	5	8	2
7	6	4	1	8	2	3	9	5
9	5	8	6	3	7	1	2	4
2	3	1	4	5	9	8	6	7
3	7	9	5	4	8	2	1	6
1	2	5	7	6	3	9	4	8
8	4	6	2	9	1	7	5	3

Puzzle # 67

4	3	2	8	1	9	7	6	5
5	1	8	4	6	7	9	3	2
7	9	6	3	2	5	4	8	1
8	2	5	7	4	3	6	1	9
9	6	7	2	5	1	8	4	3
1	4	3	6	9	8	2	5	7
2	5	1	9	8	4	3	7	6
6	7	4	1	3	2	5	9	8
3	8	9	5	7	6	1	2	4

Puzzle # 68

3	2	4	5	7	8	6	1	9
8	7	1	9	3	6	2	4	5
5	9	6	4	2	1	3	8	7
4	3	9	8	5	2	1	7	6
2	8	7	1	6	9	5	3	4
1	6	5	7	4	3	9	2	8
9	1	2	6	8	7	4	5	3
7	4	3	2	9	5	8	6	1
6	5	8	3	1	4	7	9	2

Puzzle # 69

7	1	8	5	6	9	2	4	3
2	5	4	8	7	3	9	6	1
9	6	3	4	2	1	8	5	7
1	8	5	3	4	2	7	9	6
3	7	2	9	8	6	5	1	4
6	4	9	1	5	7	3	2	8
8	9	1	6	3	5	4	7	2
4	2	6	7	9	8	1	3	5
5	3	7	2	1	4	6	8	9

Puzzle # 70

1	9	8	7	6	4	2	3	5
4	7	5	3	8	2	9	6	1
3	6	2	1	5	9	8	4	7
5	3	7	2	4	1	6	9	8
8	1	4	6	9	5	3	7	2
9	2	6	8	7	3	5	1	4
2	4	1	5	3	6	7	8	9
6	8	9	4	2	7	1	5	3
7	5	3	9	1	8	4	2	6

Puzzle # 71

2	4	7	1	6	9	8	5	3
9	3	8	4	2	5	1	6	7
6	5	1	7	8	3	2	4	9
8	6	4	5	3	7	9	1	2
3	9	2	6	4	1	7	8	5
1	7	5	8	9	2	4	3	6
7	8	3	2	1	6	5	9	4
5	1	6	9	7	4	3	2	8
4	2	9	3	5	8	6	7	1

Puzzle # 72

4	8	3	6	5	2	9	7	1
5	1	2	3	7	9	6	8	4
6	9	7	8	1	4	5	3	2
7	6	4	1	9	5	3	2	8
3	5	9	4	2	8	1	6	7
1	2	8	7	6	3	4	9	5
8	7	5	9	3	1	2	4	6
2	3	6	5	4	7	8	1	9
9	4	1	2	8	6	7	5	3

Puzzle # 73

9	2	3	7	8	4	5	6	1
6	8	7	5	1	2	3	9	4
1	4	5	9	6	3	2	8	7
5	7	2	3	9	8	1	4	6
3	6	1	4	7	5	9	2	8
4	9	8	6	2	1	7	5	3
8	5	9	1	4	7	6	3	2
2	1	6	8	3	9	4	7	5
7	3	4	2	5	6	8	1	9

Puzzle # 74

6	1	5	4	7	9	2	3	8
4	8	7	2	5	3	6	1	9
3	9	2	8	6	1	5	4	7
9	7	1	3	4	6	8	2	5
5	6	3	9	2	8	4	7	1
8	2	4	7	1	5	9	6	3
2	5	9	1	3	4	7	8	6
7	3	6	5	8	2	1	9	4
1	4	8	6	9	7	3	5	2

Puzzle # 75

5	6	9	8	7	2	1	4	3
2	8	1	4	3	6	9	5	7
3	7	4	5	9	1	2	8	6
4	3	6	1	2	8	5	7	9
1	5	2	7	4	9	6	3	8
8	9	7	6	5	3	4	2	1
7	2	8	9	1	4	3	6	5
9	4	5	3	6	7	8	1	2
6	1	3	2	8	5	7	9	4

Puzzle # 76

5	4	8	9	3	6	1	7	2
7	3	6	5	1	2	8	4	9
1	2	9	7	4	8	3	5	6
4	5	1	2	8	7	6	9	3
2	9	7	1	6	3	4	8	5
6	8	3	4	5	9	7	2	1
8	6	2	3	7	5	9	1	4
9	7	4	6	2	1	5	3	8
3	1	5	8	9	4	2	6	7

Puzzle # 77

1	9	5	6	2	4	8	3	7
8	4	7	5	1	3	9	2	6
2	3	6	7	8	9	4	1	5
6	8	4	1	7	2	5	9	3
7	2	9	3	5	8	1	6	4
3	5	1	4	9	6	2	7	8
9	7	3	8	4	1	6	5	2
4	6	2	9	3	5	7	8	1
5	1	8	2	6	7	3	4	9

Puzzle # 78

4	2	1	8	9	6	7	5	3
3	6	9	7	2	5	8	1	4
5	8	7	4	1	3	9	6	2
7	9	4	2	5	1	3	8	6
6	5	8	9	3	4	1	2	7
2	1	3	6	7	8	5	4	9
1	7	6	5	4	9	2	3	8
9	4	5	3	8	2	6	7	1
8	3	2	1	6	7	4	9	5

Puzzle # 79

7	6	4	8	1	9	2	5	3
1	2	3	5	4	6	7	8	9
8	9	5	7	3	2	1	6	4
4	1	6	9	2	3	8	7	5
2	3	7	6	5	8	9	4	1
5	8	9	4	7	1	3	2	6
3	4	8	2	9	5	6	1	7
9	7	2	1	6	4	5	3	8
6	5	1	3	8	7	4	9	2

Puzzle # 80

5	1	6	3	2	7	4	8	9
4	7	3	8	5	9	6	2	1
9	2	8	1	4	6	3	7	5
1	6	4	7	9	8	2	5	3
3	8	9	2	1	5	7	4	6
2	5	7	6	3	4	9	1	8
7	9	5	4	8	3	1	6	2
8	4	1	9	6	2	5	3	7
6	3	2	5	7	1	8	9	4

Puzzle # 81

7	3	5	6	8	2	9	4	1
8	4	9	1	3	5	6	7	2
6	1	2	9	4	7	5	8	3
2	5	4	8	7	9	1	3	6
1	8	7	2	6	3	4	5	9
9	6	3	4	5	1	8	2	7
3	7	1	5	9	4	2	6	8
5	9	8	3	2	6	7	1	4
4	2	6	7	1	8	3	9	5

Puzzle # 82

9	4	5	6	1	2	8	3	7
2	3	7	5	9	8	1	4	6
8	6	1	3	4	7	2	5	9
5	7	2	9	3	6	4	1	8
3	9	4	2	8	1	7	6	5
1	8	6	4	7	5	3	9	2
7	5	9	1	2	3	6	8	4
4	1	8	7	6	9	5	2	3
6	2	3	8	5	4	9	7	1

Puzzle # 83

1	3	2	9	5	4	7	8	6
7	8	5	2	3	6	1	4	9
9	6	4	1	8	7	2	5	3
4	9	3	6	7	1	5	2	8
5	1	7	8	2	9	6	3	4
8	2	6	5	4	3	9	1	7
3	4	9	7	1	2	8	6	5
6	5	1	4	9	8	3	7	2
2	7	8	3	6	5	4	9	1

Puzzle # 84

1	8	7	5	6	2	3	9	4
6	9	3	4	8	1	5	7	2
5	4	2	3	7	9	6	8	1
8	7	4	9	1	6	2	3	5
2	1	5	8	3	4	7	6	9
3	6	9	7	2	5	1	4	8
9	3	8	2	5	7	4	1	6
4	5	6	1	9	3	8	2	7
7	2	1	6	4	8	9	5	3

Puzzle # 85

7	6	9	2	3	1	5	4	8
5	3	4	6	9	8	1	7	2
8	1	2	5	7	4	3	6	9
6	5	8	1	4	7	2	9	3
3	9	1	8	2	6	7	5	4
4	2	7	9	5	3	8	1	6
9	8	5	4	1	2	6	3	7
2	4	3	7	6	5	9	8	1
1	7	6	3	8	9	4	2	5

Puzzle # 86

2	6	4	5	1	8	3	9	7
9	8	3	4	2	7	1	5	6
7	5	1	9	6	3	4	2	8
4	2	8	1	5	6	7	3	9
5	7	9	8	3	4	6	1	2
1	3	6	2	7	9	8	4	5
8	1	5	6	4	2	9	7	3
6	4	7	3	9	5	2	8	1
3	9	2	7	8	1	5	6	4

Puzzle # 87

3	6	4	5	9	7	2	8	1
5	7	9	8	2	1	3	6	4
8	1	2	6	4	3	9	7	5
6	5	3	1	7	2	8	4	9
9	4	8	3	5	6	7	1	2
1	2	7	9	8	4	5	3	6
4	9	5	7	6	8	1	2	3
2	8	1	4	3	9	6	5	7
7	3	6	2	1	5	4	9	8

Puzzle # 88

7	5	4	9	2	3	1	6	8
6	3	8	5	7	1	2	4	9
1	2	9	8	6	4	7	5	3
2	9	7	4	5	8	6	3	1
8	1	5	7	3	6	9	2	4
4	6	3	2	1	9	5	8	7
5	4	6	3	9	7	8	1	2
9	8	1	6	4	2	3	7	5
3	7	2	1	8	5	4	9	6

Puzzle # 89

4	9	6	1	8	7	5	3	2
5	1	2	4	9	3	8	7	6
3	7	8	6	2	5	9	4	1
6	8	5	9	3	2	4	1	7
7	3	9	5	1	4	6	2	8
1	2	4	7	6	8	3	5	9
9	4	3	8	7	1	2	6	5
8	5	7	2	4	6	1	9	3
2	6	1	3	5	9	7	8	4

Puzzle # 90

5	2	9	3	1	7	6	8	4
4	7	6	5	9	8	2	1	3
3	8	1	2	6	4	9	5	7
1	9	2	6	5	3	7	4	8
6	5	4	7	8	2	1	3	9
7	3	8	9	4	1	5	6	2
9	1	3	8	7	6	4	2	5
2	4	5	1	3	9	8	7	6
8	6	7	4	2	5	3	9	1

Puzzle # 91

9	4	3	1	6	5	7	2	8
2	5	8	4	7	9	6	3	1
7	1	6	8	3	2	5	9	4
8	7	2	6	4	1	9	5	3
5	3	1	2	9	8	4	7	6
4	6	9	3	5	7	8	1	2
6	2	7	9	1	4	3	8	5
3	8	5	7	2	6	1	4	9
1	9	4	5	8	3	2	6	7

Puzzle # 92

6	5	2	3	9	8	4	7	1
3	9	7	2	1	4	6	5	8
1	8	4	6	7	5	2	9	3
5	7	9	1	8	2	3	4	6
2	6	3	9	4	7	8	1	5
4	1	8	5	3	6	9	2	7
7	3	5	8	2	9	1	6	4
9	4	1	7	6	3	5	8	2
8	2	6	4	5	1	7	3	9

Puzzle # 93

8	6	9	5	2	7	1	4	3
1	3	7	6	8	4	5	2	9
4	5	2	3	9	1	7	8	6
7	8	5	2	3	9	6	1	4
9	4	3	1	6	8	2	5	7
2	1	6	4	7	5	3	9	8
3	7	8	9	5	2	4	6	1
6	2	4	8	1	3	9	7	5
5	9	1	7	4	6	8	3	2

Puzzle # 94

1	3	6	5	9	7	4	2	8
9	8	2	6	3	4	5	7	1
4	5	7	2	8	1	6	3	9
5	2	8	4	6	9	3	1	7
6	1	4	3	7	2	9	8	5
3	7	9	1	5	8	2	4	6
2	6	3	7	1	5	8	9	4
8	4	1	9	2	6	7	5	3
7	9	5	8	4	3	1	6	2

Puzzle # 95

2	9	3	8	1	7	6	5	4
4	5	8	9	6	2	1	3	7
6	1	7	3	4	5	9	2	8
5	4	6	7	2	9	8	1	3
7	3	2	5	8	1	4	6	9
9	8	1	6	3	4	2	7	5
3	2	9	4	5	6	7	8	1
8	6	4	1	7	3	5	9	2
1	7	5	2	9	8	3	4	6

Puzzle # 96

1	8	4	7	5	3	2	6	9
7	2	3	6	9	4	8	5	1
5	6	9	8	2	1	4	7	3
2	3	6	5	7	8	1	9	4
9	5	8	4	1	6	7	3	2
4	1	7	2	3	9	5	8	6
3	4	2	9	8	7	6	1	5
6	7	1	3	4	5	9	2	8
8	9	5	1	6	2	3	4	7

Puzzle # 97

2	7	9	1	5	3	4	6	8
1	4	3	6	9	8	2	5	7
6	5	8	2	7	4	3	9	1
7	6	5	8	3	2	1	4	9
9	3	1	4	6	5	7	8	2
8	2	4	9	1	7	6	3	5
4	9	2	3	8	1	5	7	6
5	1	6	7	4	9	8	2	3
3	8	7	5	2	6	9	1	4

Puzzle # 98

5	2	8	9	4	7	6	1	3
7	6	1	3	8	2	4	5	9
9	3	4	1	5	6	8	7	2
6	4	3	2	1	5	7	9	8
2	1	7	6	9	8	5	3	4
8	5	9	4	7	3	1	2	6
4	8	5	7	3	9	2	6	1
1	9	2	5	6	4	3	8	7
3	7	6	8	2	1	9	4	5

Puzzle # 99

6	1	8	2	3	9	7	5	4
3	2	5	4	8	7	9	6	1
7	9	4	1	5	6	3	8	2
1	7	3	6	2	8	5	4	9
5	4	2	9	7	1	6	3	8
9	8	6	5	4	3	1	2	7
2	6	1	8	9	5	4	7	3
8	3	9	7	6	4	2	1	5
4	5	7	3	1	2	8	9	6

Puzzle # 100

9	8	4	1	2	7	5	3	6
2	3	5	9	8	6	1	7	4
7	1	6	3	4	5	9	8	2
8	4	9	7	3	2	6	5	1
3	6	1	5	9	4	8	2	7
5	7	2	6	1	8	3	4	9
6	2	7	8	5	9	4	1	3
4	5	3	2	6	1	7	9	8
1	9	8	4	7	3	2	6	5

Puzzle # 101

2	9	5	8	7	3	6	1	4
4	8	3	9	1	6	5	2	7
6	7	1	5	4	2	8	9	3
3	2	8	4	5	9	1	7	6
9	6	7	2	3	1	4	5	8
5	1	4	7	6	8	9	3	2
7	3	6	1	8	5	2	4	9
8	5	2	3	9	4	7	6	1
1	4	9	6	2	7	3	8	5

Puzzle # 102

7	8	2	6	1	9	4	3	5
9	1	5	3	4	2	7	8	6
3	4	6	7	5	8	9	1	2
8	7	3	5	2	4	1	6	9
2	9	4	8	6	1	5	7	3
6	5	1	9	3	7	2	4	8
4	3	9	2	7	6	8	5	1
5	2	7	1	8	3	6	9	4
1	6	8	4	9	5	3	2	7

Puzzle # 103

3	1	6	7	8	9	5	4	2
7	9	5	4	2	1	8	3	6
8	4	2	5	6	3	1	7	9
1	2	3	9	5	8	4	6	7
5	6	7	2	1	4	9	8	3
9	8	4	6	3	7	2	1	5
4	7	1	3	9	2	6	5	8
6	3	9	8	4	5	7	2	1
2	5	8	1	7	6	3	9	4

Puzzle # 104

2	3	1	4	9	6	7	5	8
7	6	8	1	2	5	4	9	3
4	5	9	3	8	7	2	1	6
1	9	3	8	4	2	6	7	5
8	2	7	5	6	9	1	3	4
6	4	5	7	3	1	8	2	9
9	8	2	6	7	3	5	4	1
3	1	4	2	5	8	9	6	7
5	7	6	9	1	4	3	8	2

Puzzle # 105

5	3	9	7	4	2	1	8	6
2	6	8	5	3	1	7	9	4
7	4	1	6	8	9	3	5	2
1	8	7	3	2	4	5	6	9
3	2	6	9	1	5	4	7	8
4	9	5	8	7	6	2	1	3
9	7	3	4	5	8	6	2	1
8	5	2	1	6	3	9	4	7
6	1	4	2	9	7	8	3	5

Puzzle # 106

2	3	7	8	9	5	1	6	4
6	5	4	7	3	1	8	9	2
9	8	1	4	2	6	5	7	3
5	4	2	1	6	3	7	8	9
8	1	9	5	4	7	3	2	6
7	6	3	2	8	9	4	1	5
4	2	5	9	1	8	6	3	7
1	7	6	3	5	2	9	4	8
3	9	8	6	7	4	2	5	1

Puzzle # 107

3	9	5	1	7	6	8	2	4
8	4	2	5	3	9	7	1	6
6	7	1	2	4	8	3	9	5
7	1	9	6	8	5	4	3	2
5	3	6	4	1	2	9	8	7
4	2	8	3	9	7	5	6	1
2	6	3	8	5	4	1	7	9
1	5	7	9	6	3	2	4	8
9	8	4	7	2	1	6	5	3

Puzzle # 108

5	7	9	1	4	2	6	3	8
6	1	4	3	8	9	7	5	2
8	2	3	7	5	6	4	9	1
7	8	2	4	3	1	5	6	9
9	4	5	2	6	8	1	7	3
3	6	1	9	7	5	2	8	4
4	5	8	6	2	3	9	1	7
1	3	7	5	9	4	8	2	6
2	9	6	8	1	7	3	4	5

Puzzle # 109

5	3	7	1	6	9	2	8	4
6	9	1	2	8	4	3	5	7
2	8	4	7	5	3	9	1	6
7	1	8	3	2	5	6	4	9
4	5	3	6	9	8	1	7	2
9	6	2	4	7	1	8	3	5
3	7	6	8	4	2	5	9	1
8	4	9	5	1	6	7	2	3
1	2	5	9	3	7	4	6	8

Puzzle # 110

5	6	8	1	7	9	4	3	2
2	7	4	5	6	3	1	8	9
1	9	3	8	2	4	5	6	7
4	2	5	9	8	6	7	1	3
9	8	7	3	1	2	6	5	4
6	3	1	4	5	7	9	2	8
3	5	6	7	9	8	2	4	1
8	1	9	2	4	5	3	7	6
7	4	2	6	3	1	8	9	5

Puzzle # 111

1	7	3	6	8	9	4	5	2
4	2	8	3	7	5	6	9	1
5	9	6	1	2	4	7	3	8
9	8	5	7	3	1	2	4	6
6	4	7	2	9	8	5	1	3
3	1	2	5	4	6	8	7	9
8	6	4	9	1	7	3	2	5
7	3	1	8	5	2	9	6	4
2	5	9	4	6	3	1	8	7

Puzzle # 112

6	9	4	5	2	7	3	1	8
3	1	5	6	4	8	9	2	7
8	7	2	3	1	9	5	6	4
5	3	1	4	8	6	2	7	9
4	6	9	2	7	1	8	5	3
7	2	8	9	3	5	6	4	1
2	8	6	7	9	4	1	3	5
1	5	7	8	6	3	4	9	2
9	4	3	1	5	2	7	8	6

Puzzle # 113

2	6	8	9	4	5	7	1	3
5	9	4	7	1	3	8	6	2
3	7	1	6	2	8	4	5	9
7	4	9	2	5	1	3	8	6
1	3	6	4	8	9	5	2	7
8	5	2	3	6	7	9	4	1
9	1	5	8	7	6	2	3	4
4	8	3	1	9	2	6	7	5
6	2	7	5	3	4	1	9	8

Puzzle # 114

6	1	7	9	5	4	3	2	8
8	3	4	7	6	2	1	5	9
9	2	5	3	8	1	7	6	4
1	6	2	5	3	9	4	8	7
4	7	3	1	2	8	5	9	6
5	8	9	4	7	6	2	3	1
7	4	6	2	9	3	8	1	5
3	5	8	6	1	7	9	4	2
2	9	1	8	4	5	6	7	3

Puzzle # 115

9	3	2	8	1	7	4	6	5
1	6	4	2	3	5	7	8	9
8	7	5	9	4	6	1	2	3
5	2	9	6	7	3	8	4	1
3	4	1	5	2	8	6	9	7
7	8	6	1	9	4	5	3	2
4	1	8	3	5	2	9	7	6
6	5	3	7	8	9	2	1	4
2	9	7	4	6	1	3	5	8

Puzzle # 116

1	9	6	5	8	2	4	3	7
8	7	5	3	4	6	1	9	2
4	2	3	1	7	9	6	5	8
9	1	7	4	3	8	5	2	6
5	6	8	9	2	1	7	4	3
3	4	2	7	6	5	8	1	9
7	3	1	8	9	4	2	6	5
6	5	9	2	1	7	3	8	4
2	8	4	6	5	3	9	7	1

Puzzle # 117

6	1	4	5	8	7	9	3	2
5	9	8	1	2	3	6	4	7
3	2	7	9	6	4	5	1	8
9	8	2	3	7	5	1	6	4
7	3	1	4	9	6	2	8	5
4	6	5	8	1	2	3	7	9
1	4	9	6	5	8	7	2	3
8	7	6	2	3	9	4	5	1
2	5	3	7	4	1	8	9	6

Puzzle # 118

2	8	5	4	9	7	3	6	1
6	3	7	2	8	1	9	4	5
1	4	9	6	5	3	8	2	7
4	9	6	5	1	2	7	3	8
5	2	1	7	3	8	4	9	6
3	7	8	9	6	4	5	1	2
7	6	4	3	2	5	1	8	9
9	1	3	8	7	6	2	5	4
8	5	2	1	4	9	6	7	3

Puzzle # 119

5	6	9	3	7	8	1	2	4
3	4	8	2	6	1	5	7	9
1	2	7	4	9	5	6	8	3
6	7	4	5	1	3	8	9	2
8	1	5	9	4	2	3	6	7
2	9	3	7	8	6	4	1	5
9	3	1	6	5	7	2	4	8
4	8	2	1	3	9	7	5	6
7	5	6	8	2	4	9	3	1

Puzzle # 120

4	8	9	2	6	7	3	5	1
5	2	7	8	1	3	4	6	9
6	3	1	4	5	9	8	2	7
9	4	8	3	2	6	7	1	5
2	1	3	5	7	4	6	9	8
7	5	6	9	8	1	2	4	3
8	6	4	1	3	5	9	7	2
1	9	2	7	4	8	5	3	6
3	7	5	6	9	2	1	8	4

Puzzle # 121

8	3	2	6	4	7	9	1	5
6	7	9	5	3	1	2	8	4
1	5	4	9	2	8	6	7	3
7	1	8	4	5	9	3	2	6
9	2	5	8	6	3	7	4	1
3	4	6	1	7	2	5	9	8
2	8	3	7	1	5	4	6	9
5	6	1	2	9	4	8	3	7
4	9	7	3	8	6	1	5	2

Puzzle # 122

9	3	1	5	4	7	6	2	8
5	7	4	8	6	2	9	1	3
2	8	6	3	1	9	7	5	4
4	9	7	6	2	8	5	3	1
6	5	3	1	7	4	8	9	2
1	2	8	9	3	5	4	7	6
7	4	9	2	8	3	1	6	5
3	6	5	4	9	1	2	8	7
8	1	2	7	5	6	3	4	9

Puzzle # 123

1	6	3	7	8	4	5	9	2
7	9	8	2	6	5	4	1	3
2	4	5	9	1	3	7	6	8
5	8	2	3	4	6	1	7	9
9	3	7	1	5	2	6	8	4
6	1	4	8	9	7	3	2	5
4	5	9	6	7	8	2	3	1
3	7	1	4	2	9	8	5	6
8	2	6	5	3	1	9	4	7

Puzzle # 124

1	8	5	9	7	4	2	6	3
4	7	2	6	3	5	8	1	9
6	3	9	2	8	1	4	5	7
8	2	1	5	4	7	3	9	6
9	4	3	8	1	6	5	7	2
5	6	7	3	2	9	1	4	8
3	1	6	7	5	8	9	2	4
2	9	4	1	6	3	7	8	5
7	5	8	4	9	2	6	3	1

Puzzle # 125

1	4	5	9	7	2	8	3	6
3	2	9	6	5	8	4	1	7
8	7	6	4	1	3	9	2	5
9	8	7	1	3	4	6	5	2
6	5	3	8	2	7	1	9	4
4	1	2	5	6	9	3	7	8
5	3	4	2	9	6	7	8	1
2	9	8	7	4	1	5	6	3
7	6	1	3	8	5	2	4	9

Puzzle # 126

7	9	8	3	6	4	1	5	2
3	4	5	7	2	1	6	8	9
1	6	2	5	8	9	7	3	4
6	2	1	9	3	8	4	7	5
4	8	7	2	5	6	3	9	1
5	3	9	1	4	7	2	6	8
9	7	3	8	1	2	5	4	6
2	5	6	4	9	3	8	1	7
8	1	4	6	7	5	9	2	3

Puzzle # 127

8	1	3	4	6	5	7	2	9
5	4	2	1	7	9	3	8	6
7	6	9	2	3	8	4	1	5
9	7	8	6	1	4	5	3	2
6	5	4	3	8	2	9	7	1
3	2	1	5	9	7	8	6	4
2	8	5	7	4	1	6	9	3
1	9	6	8	5	3	2	4	7
4	3	7	9	2	6	1	5	8

Puzzle # 128

2	9	5	7	1	3	8	6	4
1	3	6	4	2	8	5	7	9
8	7	4	6	5	9	2	1	3
5	2	3	9	6	4	1	8	7
7	8	1	5	3	2	9	4	6
4	6	9	1	8	7	3	2	5
3	4	7	8	9	1	6	5	2
9	5	8	2	4	6	7	3	1
6	1	2	3	7	5	4	9	8

Puzzle # 129

7	1	6	5	8	9	2	3	4
8	3	5	1	4	2	9	6	7
4	2	9	3	7	6	8	1	5
3	7	1	6	5	8	4	9	2
9	4	8	2	3	7	6	5	1
6	5	2	4	9	1	7	8	3
2	6	4	9	1	3	5	7	8
5	8	3	7	6	4	1	2	9
1	9	7	8	2	5	3	4	6

Puzzle # 130

1	3	7	6	4	5	2	8	9
8	2	5	9	3	1	6	7	4
6	4	9	7	8	2	1	3	5
4	1	2	8	6	7	9	5	3
9	7	6	4	5	3	8	1	2
3	5	8	1	2	9	4	6	7
2	6	3	5	9	8	7	4	1
7	9	4	3	1	6	5	2	8
5	8	1	2	7	4	3	9	6

Puzzle # 131

2	1	9	7	5	8	6	4	3
6	3	7	9	4	1	8	2	5
5	4	8	6	2	3	1	7	9
8	9	3	1	7	5	2	6	4
1	2	6	3	9	4	7	5	8
7	5	4	2	8	6	9	3	1
3	8	1	5	6	2	4	9	7
4	7	2	8	3	9	5	1	6
9	6	5	4	1	7	3	8	2

Puzzle # 132

1	9	3	2	6	8	4	7	5
8	2	7	3	5	4	6	9	1
4	6	5	1	9	7	3	2	8
3	8	9	5	1	2	7	4	6
6	7	1	8	4	3	9	5	2
2	5	4	6	7	9	8	1	3
5	4	8	7	3	1	2	6	9
7	1	2	9	8	6	5	3	4
9	3	6	4	2	5	1	8	7

Puzzle # 133

8	7	6	3	4	2	9	1	5
5	9	3	6	1	8	2	7	4
1	2	4	7	5	9	8	3	6
6	1	5	8	7	3	4	2	9
2	3	9	4	6	5	7	8	1
7	4	8	9	2	1	6	5	3
3	6	1	2	8	4	5	9	7
4	5	2	1	9	7	3	6	8
9	8	7	5	3	6	1	4	2

Puzzle # 134

9	7	2	3	4	5	1	8	6
6	3	4	1	8	7	2	9	5
1	5	8	6	2	9	4	7	3
4	2	5	7	6	1	8	3	9
8	9	6	2	5	3	7	4	1
7	1	3	4	9	8	6	5	2
2	8	1	5	3	4	9	6	7
3	4	7	9	1	6	5	2	8
5	6	9	8	7	2	3	1	4

Puzzle # 135

5	3	7	6	9	2	1	8	4
8	1	2	3	4	5	7	9	6
6	9	4	1	8	7	5	2	3
2	8	6	9	5	1	3	4	7
3	7	1	8	6	4	9	5	2
4	5	9	7	2	3	8	6	1
7	4	8	5	1	6	2	3	9
1	6	5	2	3	9	4	7	8
9	2	3	4	7	8	6	1	5

Puzzle # 136

9	6	8	7	2	1	5	4	3
7	2	3	9	5	4	8	1	6
1	5	4	3	8	6	7	2	9
8	4	1	6	9	2	3	7	5
5	3	2	8	1	7	9	6	4
6	9	7	5	4	3	1	8	2
4	1	5	2	3	8	6	9	7
2	7	9	1	6	5	4	3	8
3	8	6	4	7	9	2	5	1

Puzzle # 137

3	5	2	7	6	1	4	8	9
7	1	6	9	4	8	5	3	2
4	8	9	2	5	3	1	7	6
1	6	8	4	2	9	3	5	7
2	9	4	5	3	7	6	1	8
5	7	3	8	1	6	9	2	4
8	3	5	6	7	4	2	9	1
9	4	1	3	8	2	7	6	5
6	2	7	1	9	5	8	4	3

Puzzle # 138

9	6	1	3	4	8	5	7	2
2	4	5	9	6	7	1	3	8
8	7	3	1	2	5	4	9	6
6	2	7	8	1	4	3	5	9
3	9	4	5	7	6	2	8	1
5	1	8	2	3	9	6	4	7
7	3	9	6	5	2	8	1	4
4	5	6	7	8	1	9	2	3
1	8	2	4	9	3	7	6	5

Puzzle # 139

5	8	9	1	7	3	4	2	6
6	3	1	2	4	8	9	5	7
4	7	2	5	9	6	1	3	8
2	6	3	7	1	4	5	8	9
8	5	4	9	3	2	7	6	1
1	9	7	6	8	5	3	4	2
9	2	8	3	5	1	6	7	4
3	1	6	4	2	7	8	9	5
7	4	5	8	6	9	2	1	3

Puzzle # 140

7	5	6	4	2	9	1	3	8
9	8	3	6	1	7	2	4	5
1	2	4	5	3	8	6	9	7
8	4	9	3	6	5	7	1	2
5	3	7	2	8	1	4	6	9
6	1	2	7	9	4	5	8	3
2	6	5	8	4	3	9	7	1
3	7	1	9	5	6	8	2	4
4	9	8	1	7	2	3	5	6

Puzzle # 141

1	3	2	9	8	4	7	6	5
4	8	7	5	2	6	1	3	9
5	6	9	7	3	1	8	4	2
8	7	5	4	9	3	2	1	6
3	9	4	1	6	2	5	7	8
6	2	1	8	5	7	3	9	4
9	4	8	3	7	5	6	2	1
2	5	3	6	1	9	4	8	7
7	1	6	2	4	8	9	5	3

Puzzle # 142

8	4	3	9	7	5	2	6	1
5	2	1	8	3	6	4	7	9
6	7	9	2	4	1	8	3	5
9	1	4	3	2	7	5	8	6
2	3	8	5	6	9	7	1	4
7	6	5	1	8	4	9	2	3
3	5	7	4	1	2	6	9	8
4	8	2	6	9	3	1	5	7
1	9	6	7	5	8	3	4	2

Puzzle # 143

9	2	6	4	5	3	7	8	1
3	4	1	7	8	9	6	2	5
7	5	8	2	6	1	9	4	3
5	9	7	8	1	2	3	6	4
6	1	2	9	3	4	5	7	8
8	3	4	6	7	5	2	1	9
1	8	5	3	2	6	4	9	7
2	7	9	5	4	8	1	3	6
4	6	3	1	9	7	8	5	2

Puzzle # 144

2	3	5	1	4	6	7	9	8
6	9	8	7	5	3	1	2	4
7	4	1	8	9	2	5	3	6
3	7	9	4	6	1	8	5	2
1	5	2	9	7	8	6	4	3
4	8	6	2	3	5	9	1	7
9	6	7	5	2	4	3	8	1
8	2	3	6	1	9	4	7	5
5	1	4	3	8	7	2	6	9

Puzzle # 145

7	4	5	2	3	9	8	1	6
1	2	3	8	6	7	9	5	4
8	9	6	5	1	4	2	7	3
9	8	2	7	5	6	3	4	1
5	6	4	1	8	3	7	9	2
3	7	1	9	4	2	5	6	8
4	5	7	6	2	8	1	3	9
6	1	8	3	9	5	4	2	7
2	3	9	4	7	1	6	8	5

Puzzle # 146

7	6	1	2	8	9	5	4	3
8	2	5	1	3	4	9	6	7
3	9	4	7	6	5	1	8	2
1	3	7	4	9	8	6	2	5
2	4	8	6	5	1	3	7	9
9	5	6	3	2	7	4	1	8
5	1	2	9	7	6	8	3	4
4	7	9	8	1	3	2	5	6
6	8	3	5	4	2	7	9	1

Puzzle # 147

2	1	6	5	8	4	7	9	3
8	3	9	7	6	1	4	5	2
4	7	5	3	9	2	8	1	6
1	9	2	6	3	7	5	8	4
5	8	7	2	4	9	3	6	1
3	6	4	1	5	8	2	7	9
9	2	1	4	7	5	6	3	8
6	5	8	9	2	3	1	4	7
7	4	3	8	1	6	9	2	5

Puzzle # 148

9	7	8	2	3	6	1	5	4
1	2	5	7	9	4	6	8	3
6	4	3	8	1	5	9	2	7
2	3	4	9	6	7	5	1	8
8	1	6	4	5	3	7	9	2
7	5	9	1	2	8	4	3	6
3	6	7	5	8	9	2	4	1
5	8	1	6	4	2	3	7	9
4	9	2	3	7	1	8	6	5

Puzzle # 149

9	4	1	6	7	2	8	5	3
6	2	3	8	5	4	9	7	1
5	8	7	3	9	1	2	4	6
1	6	5	2	3	9	4	8	7
4	7	9	5	6	8	3	1	2
2	3	8	4	1	7	5	6	9
8	9	4	1	2	6	7	3	5
3	1	2	7	8	5	6	9	4
7	5	6	9	4	3	1	2	8

Puzzle # 150

1	4	7	5	9	3	8	2	6
5	2	9	7	8	6	1	4	3
6	3	8	2	4	1	9	5	7
3	1	5	9	6	7	4	8	2
4	8	6	1	2	5	3	7	9
7	9	2	4	3	8	6	1	5
8	6	1	3	5	2	7	9	4
9	5	3	8	7	4	2	6	1
2	7	4	6	1	9	5	3	8

Puzzle # 151

6	9	3	5	4	2	8	7	1
2	8	5	7	6	1	3	9	4
7	4	1	3	9	8	6	5	2
4	2	7	1	3	9	5	8	6
8	5	9	6	2	7	1	4	3
3	1	6	8	5	4	7	2	9
9	6	8	2	7	3	4	1	5
1	3	4	9	8	5	2	6	7
5	7	2	4	1	6	9	3	8

Puzzle # 152

1	3	7	4	8	5	6	9	2
2	4	8	9	7	6	3	1	5
9	6	5	2	3	1	7	4	8
5	7	9	6	2	3	4	8	1
8	2	3	5	1	4	9	7	6
4	1	6	7	9	8	2	5	3
3	5	2	8	4	7	1	6	9
6	9	4	1	5	2	8	3	7
7	8	1	3	6	9	5	2	4

Puzzle # 153

1	8	9	3	7	5	6	2	4
2	7	4	1	9	6	3	5	8
6	3	5	4	2	8	7	1	9
4	2	8	9	5	7	1	3	6
7	9	6	8	1	3	2	4	5
5	1	3	6	4	2	9	8	7
8	4	2	7	6	1	5	9	3
9	5	7	2	3	4	8	6	1
3	6	1	5	8	9	4	7	2

Puzzle # 154

1	2	6	4	7	3	5	9	8
8	9	5	6	1	2	3	7	4
7	3	4	5	8	9	2	1	6
6	7	2	8	3	5	9	4	1
4	1	3	9	2	7	6	8	5
9	5	8	1	4	6	7	3	2
5	8	9	7	6	1	4	2	3
3	4	7	2	5	8	1	6	9
2	6	1	3	9	4	8	5	7

Puzzle # 155

5	4	8	3	2	1	6	7	9
9	2	6	4	7	5	3	8	1
7	3	1	9	8	6	5	2	4
8	5	9	6	4	3	2	1	7
1	6	4	7	5	2	9	3	8
2	7	3	8	1	9	4	5	6
4	1	5	2	6	8	7	9	3
3	8	7	5	9	4	1	6	2
6	9	2	1	3	7	8	4	5

Puzzle # 156

3	4	2	8	7	9	5	1	6
1	7	9	5	3	6	8	2	4
8	6	5	1	4	2	7	9	3
4	2	6	3	1	7	9	5	8
9	1	3	2	8	5	6	4	7
5	8	7	6	9	4	1	3	2
6	9	4	7	2	1	3	8	5
2	5	8	9	6	3	4	7	1
7	3	1	4	5	8	2	6	9

Puzzle # 157

1	2	5	4	6	8	7	9	3
9	7	4	1	3	2	6	8	5
6	3	8	9	5	7	2	1	4
2	8	3	5	7	1	9	4	6
4	1	7	6	8	9	3	5	2
5	9	6	3	2	4	1	7	8
3	6	9	7	4	5	8	2	1
7	4	2	8	1	3	5	6	9
8	5	1	2	9	6	4	3	7

Puzzle # 158

2	4	3	5	9	8	7	6	1
1	7	8	3	4	6	5	2	9
9	5	6	1	2	7	8	3	4
5	2	4	6	1	9	3	8	7
3	6	7	4	8	2	9	1	5
8	9	1	7	3	5	6	4	2
4	3	9	8	7	1	2	5	6
6	1	2	9	5	3	4	7	8
7	8	5	2	6	4	1	9	3

Puzzle # 159

9	3	4	5	8	6	1	7	2
2	5	1	7	9	3	6	4	8
6	7	8	1	4	2	9	3	5
8	6	3	2	1	5	4	9	7
4	1	9	3	7	8	2	5	6
7	2	5	9	6	4	3	8	1
5	8	6	4	3	1	7	2	9
3	9	2	6	5	7	8	1	4
1	4	7	8	2	9	5	6	3

Puzzle # 160

2	9	3	7	4	5	8	6	1
4	6	7	8	1	2	9	3	5
8	1	5	9	3	6	4	2	7
3	2	9	1	5	8	7	4	6
5	4	1	6	7	9	2	8	3
7	8	6	3	2	4	5	1	9
6	7	4	5	8	1	3	9	2
1	3	8	2	9	7	6	5	4
9	5	2	4	6	3	1	7	8

Puzzle # 161

5	9	8	3	4	6	2	1	7
3	4	6	1	2	7	8	9	5
2	7	1	5	8	9	4	3	6
8	6	5	2	9	3	1	7	4
1	3	7	8	6	4	9	5	2
9	2	4	7	1	5	3	6	8
7	8	9	6	3	2	5	4	1
4	5	2	9	7	1	6	8	3
6	1	3	4	5	8	7	2	9

Puzzle # 162

5	7	2	1	6	4	8	9	3
4	9	3	5	8	7	2	1	6
1	8	6	3	2	9	5	7	4
6	4	1	2	5	3	9	8	7
8	3	9	7	1	6	4	2	5
7	2	5	4	9	8	6	3	1
2	5	7	8	4	1	3	6	9
3	6	8	9	7	5	1	4	2
9	1	4	6	3	2	7	5	8

Puzzle # 163

9	3	8	1	4	7	2	5	6
5	2	1	6	3	9	8	7	4
7	6	4	2	8	5	3	1	9
8	5	9	7	6	3	4	2	1
4	7	3	5	2	1	9	6	8
6	1	2	4	9	8	5	3	7
1	8	5	3	7	4	6	9	2
3	4	6	9	1	2	7	8	5
2	9	7	8	5	6	1	4	3

Puzzle # 164

1	7	2	6	5	4	8	9	3
5	9	3	7	8	2	4	1	6
6	8	4	1	9	3	7	2	5
3	2	8	4	6	5	9	7	1
7	6	5	2	1	9	3	8	4
4	1	9	3	7	8	6	5	2
8	5	6	9	4	1	2	3	7
9	3	7	5	2	6	1	4	8
2	4	1	8	3	7	5	6	9

Puzzle # 165

2	5	6	4	9	8	1	7	3
7	3	1	6	2	5	4	8	9
9	4	8	7	3	1	6	5	2
6	1	9	3	4	7	8	2	5
3	2	5	9	8	6	7	1	4
4	8	7	5	1	2	3	9	6
5	7	2	1	6	4	9	3	8
8	6	3	2	7	9	5	4	1
1	9	4	8	5	3	2	6	7

Puzzle # 166

1	4	9	3	8	6	5	2	7
6	3	2	7	1	5	4	8	9
5	7	8	4	2	9	3	6	1
4	2	7	9	6	1	8	5	3
3	8	6	2	5	7	1	9	4
9	1	5	8	4	3	6	7	2
7	5	3	1	9	8	2	4	6
8	9	4	6	3	2	7	1	5
2	6	1	5	7	4	9	3	8

Puzzle # 167

9	5	8	3	2	1	6	7	4
6	2	4	9	8	7	1	5	3
3	1	7	6	4	5	2	9	8
7	4	3	5	1	2	8	6	9
1	6	9	8	7	3	5	4	2
5	8	2	4	6	9	7	3	1
8	9	1	7	3	6	4	2	5
2	7	5	1	9	4	3	8	6
4	3	6	2	5	8	9	1	7

Puzzle # 168

8	4	6	2	7	5	1	9	3
2	9	7	1	3	6	4	8	5
1	5	3	9	8	4	2	7	6
4	6	9	3	2	8	5	1	7
7	3	8	5	6	1	9	4	2
5	2	1	4	9	7	6	3	8
9	8	5	7	1	2	3	6	4
3	7	4	6	5	9	8	2	1
6	1	2	8	4	3	7	5	9

Puzzle # 169

3	2	7	6	8	1	5	4	9
6	5	1	4	3	9	7	8	2
8	9	4	5	7	2	1	3	6
4	6	9	7	5	8	2	1	3
5	8	2	1	9	3	6	7	4
1	7	3	2	6	4	8	9	5
2	3	6	8	4	7	9	5	1
7	4	5	9	1	6	3	2	8
9	1	8	3	2	5	4	6	7

Puzzle # 170

3	1	4	8	7	6	2	5	9
6	8	9	4	2	5	7	3	1
2	7	5	3	9	1	4	6	8
9	2	1	7	3	8	5	4	6
7	6	8	1	5	4	9	2	3
4	5	3	9	6	2	1	8	7
8	9	2	6	4	7	3	1	5
5	3	6	2	1	9	8	7	4
1	4	7	5	8	3	6	9	2

Puzzle # 171

9	1	6	4	3	2	5	8	7
7	2	4	6	5	8	1	9	3
3	5	8	7	1	9	2	6	4
1	6	5	3	8	4	9	7	2
4	7	3	9	2	1	6	5	8
2	8	9	5	7	6	3	4	1
6	3	2	8	9	7	4	1	5
5	9	7	1	4	3	8	2	6
8	4	1	2	6	5	7	3	9

Puzzle # 172

9	7	5	2	1	8	4	6	3
4	1	3	9	6	5	2	7	8
6	8	2	4	3	7	5	1	9
5	6	4	8	9	3	7	2	1
8	3	7	1	2	4	6	9	5
2	9	1	5	7	6	8	3	4
7	5	6	3	4	1	9	8	2
3	4	9	6	8	2	1	5	7
1	2	8	7	5	9	3	4	6

Puzzle # 173

1	3	6	2	4	8	5	9	7
5	8	7	1	9	6	2	4	3
2	9	4	5	7	3	6	1	8
7	1	9	3	6	2	4	8	5
8	6	2	4	5	9	3	7	1
4	5	3	7	8	1	9	2	6
3	2	8	9	1	5	7	6	4
6	4	5	8	2	7	1	3	9
9	7	1	6	3	4	8	5	2

Puzzle # 174

8	9	3	4	5	1	6	2	7
4	6	5	2	9	7	8	3	1
1	2	7	8	3	6	4	5	9
7	3	6	5	2	9	1	8	4
2	5	8	1	7	4	3	9	6
9	1	4	3	6	8	2	7	5
3	4	9	6	8	5	7	1	2
6	7	2	9	1	3	5	4	8
5	8	1	7	4	2	9	6	3

Puzzle # 175

6	5	1	8	9	4	3	2	7
7	8	4	5	2	3	6	9	1
2	9	3	6	7	1	8	5	4
8	3	5	7	4	2	1	6	9
4	6	9	3	1	5	7	8	2
1	7	2	9	6	8	4	3	5
9	2	7	4	3	6	5	1	8
3	4	8	1	5	9	2	7	6
5	1	6	2	8	7	9	4	3

Puzzle # 176

4	6	8	1	5	2	3	9	7
3	1	7	9	4	8	6	2	5
5	9	2	3	6	7	1	8	4
8	5	1	6	2	9	7	4	3
7	3	6	8	1	4	2	5	9
2	4	9	5	7	3	8	1	6
6	8	4	2	3	5	9	7	1
1	2	5	7	9	6	4	3	8
9	7	3	4	8	1	5	6	2

Puzzle # 177

1	7	6	5	2	8	3	9	4
4	5	8	3	1	9	7	6	2
3	9	2	4	7	6	1	5	8
9	4	5	1	8	7	2	3	6
2	8	1	6	3	4	9	7	5
7	6	3	2	9	5	4	8	1
6	1	7	8	4	3	5	2	9
5	3	4	9	6	2	8	1	7
8	2	9	7	5	1	6	4	3

Puzzle # 178

4	2	8	5	7	9	1	6	3
1	5	7	6	3	8	4	2	9
9	3	6	2	4	1	7	8	5
2	9	4	8	6	7	3	5	1
8	6	3	1	9	5	2	7	4
5	7	1	4	2	3	6	9	8
3	8	9	7	1	2	5	4	6
6	1	2	9	5	4	8	3	7
7	4	5	3	8	6	9	1	2

Puzzle # 179

2	8	9	5	3	4	1	7	6
3	6	7	2	8	1	5	9	4
5	4	1	7	9	6	2	8	3
9	2	3	6	7	5	4	1	8
7	1	6	8	4	9	3	2	5
4	5	8	3	1	2	7	6	9
6	7	2	9	5	3	8	4	1
8	3	4	1	6	7	9	5	2
1	9	5	4	2	8	6	3	7

Puzzle # 180

9	2	1	5	8	7	4	6	3
4	6	3	2	1	9	8	7	5
7	5	8	3	4	6	1	2	9
3	1	9	6	2	8	7	5	4
5	4	6	7	9	1	2	3	8
2	8	7	4	5	3	6	9	1
1	9	2	8	7	5	3	4	6
8	3	4	9	6	2	5	1	7
6	7	5	1	3	4	9	8	2

Puzzle # 181

2	9	5	3	8	4	6	7	1
1	4	7	9	5	6	3	2	8
6	8	3	2	1	7	9	5	4
8	5	6	4	7	3	1	9	2
7	2	4	1	9	5	8	3	6
3	1	9	6	2	8	7	4	5
9	3	2	8	4	1	5	6	7
4	7	1	5	6	9	2	8	3
5	6	8	7	3	2	4	1	9

Puzzle # 182

8	9	5	1	6	2	3	4	7
1	4	6	7	3	5	2	9	8
3	7	2	4	9	8	1	5	6
2	3	7	5	8	1	4	6	9
9	8	4	3	7	6	5	1	2
5	6	1	2	4	9	7	8	3
6	1	3	9	5	7	8	2	4
7	2	9	8	1	4	6	3	5
4	5	8	6	2	3	9	7	1

Puzzle # 183

3	1	6	7	8	9	5	4	2
4	7	8	3	2	5	6	1	9
9	5	2	1	6	4	3	8	7
8	6	7	9	3	1	2	5	4
5	2	3	6	4	7	8	9	1
1	4	9	2	5	8	7	6	3
7	8	1	5	9	3	4	2	6
2	9	4	8	7	6	1	3	5
6	3	5	4	1	2	9	7	8

Puzzle # 184

3	4	2	5	7	8	9	1	6
1	7	6	4	3	9	2	8	5
8	9	5	1	6	2	4	7	3
4	2	1	3	5	7	6	9	8
9	5	3	8	2	6	7	4	1
7	6	8	9	1	4	5	3	2
2	1	9	7	8	5	3	6	4
6	3	4	2	9	1	8	5	7
5	8	7	6	4	3	1	2	9

Puzzle # 185

7	4	5	3	1	9	2	6	8
6	2	9	7	5	8	1	4	3
1	3	8	4	6	2	9	7	5
4	1	7	2	9	5	8	3	6
8	5	6	1	4	3	7	2	9
3	9	2	8	7	6	4	5	1
2	6	1	9	3	7	5	8	4
5	7	4	6	8	1	3	9	2
9	8	3	5	2	4	6	1	7

Puzzle # 186

1	4	3	8	5	7	2	6	9
5	2	7	9	6	1	8	4	3
8	6	9	2	4	3	7	1	5
4	5	1	7	9	6	3	2	8
3	9	2	5	1	8	4	7	6
6	7	8	4	3	2	5	9	1
7	1	5	6	8	4	9	3	2
9	3	4	1	2	5	6	8	7
2	8	6	3	7	9	1	5	4

Puzzle # 187

6	8	2	4	3	1	9	5	7
3	1	7	9	5	2	8	6	4
9	5	4	6	8	7	2	3	1
5	3	6	8	1	9	4	7	2
7	4	9	5	2	6	3	1	8
8	2	1	3	7	4	5	9	6
1	9	8	7	4	5	6	2	3
2	6	3	1	9	8	7	4	5
4	7	5	2	6	3	1	8	9

Puzzle # 188

8	2	1	9	7	4	5	3	6
3	6	4	5	1	8	9	2	7
9	5	7	3	2	6	1	4	8
6	1	2	4	8	5	3	7	9
7	9	8	1	6	3	4	5	2
4	3	5	7	9	2	8	6	1
5	8	6	2	3	9	7	1	4
2	7	3	8	4	1	6	9	5
1	4	9	6	5	7	2	8	3